'Doctor, There's Something Wrong with My Guts!'

A Symptomatic Guide to Gastroenterology

'Doctor, There's Something Wrong with My Guts!'

A Symptomatic Guide to Gastroenterology

edited by

ROY POUNDER MD, MRCP
Consultant Physician and Gastroenterologist,
The Royal Free Hospital, London

Picture editor

ALBERTO SANTANA MD
Research Fellow, Academic Department of Medicine,
The Royal Free Hospital, London

Produced by Smith Kline & French Laboratories Limited
as a service to continuing medical education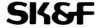

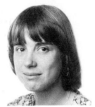

V. Alun Jones BA, MB, BChir
Research Fellow, Department of Gastroenterology, Addenbrooke's Hospital, Cambridge

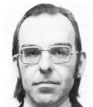

Malcolm C. Bateson MD, MRCP
Consultant Physician and Specialist in Gastroenterology, Bishop Auckland General Hospital, County Durham

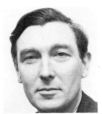

John Bull MRCP, MRCS
Physician, Worthing, West Sussex

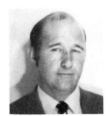

K.G. Burnand MS, FRCS
Assistant Director, Surgical Unit, St Thomas's Hospital, London

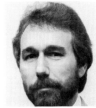

Russell Cowan MD, MRCP
Consultant Physician, Essex County Hospital, Colchester, Essex

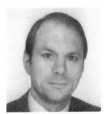

P.D. Fairclough MD, MRCP
Consultant Physician and Gastroenterologist, St Bartholomew's Hospital, London

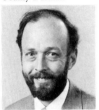

Brian Gazzard MA, MD, FRCP
Consultant Physician, St Stephen's Hospital, London

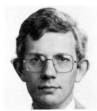

Ian Gilmore MA, MD, MRCP
Consultant Physician and Gastroenterologist, Royal Liverpool and Broadgreen Hospital, Liverpool

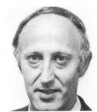

Michael Goodman MRCP
Consultant Physician, Bury Area Health Authority, Lancashire

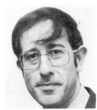

Stuart R. Gould BSc, MD, MRCP
Consultant Physician and Gastroenterologist, Epsom District Hospital, Surrey

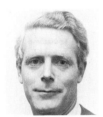

Michael D. Hellier MA, MD, FRCP
Consultant Physician, Princess Margaret Hospital, Swindon, Wiltshire

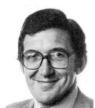

J.O. Hunter MA, MD
Consultant Physician, Addenbrooke's Hospital, Cambridge

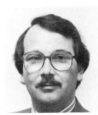

Stephen P. Kane MA, BM, MRCP
Consultant Physician, West Middlesex University Hospital, Isleworth, Middlesex

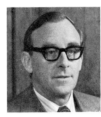

Graeme D. Kerr FRCP, FRACP
Consultant Physician and Gastroenterologist, Royal Shrewsbury Hospital, Shropshire

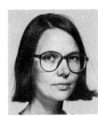

Christine Lee MA, MRCP
Senior Registrar in Haematology, Royal Free Hospital, London

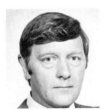

Adam Lewis FRCS
Consultant Surgeon, Royal Free Hospital, London

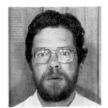

W.J.S. Ruddell MD
Consultant Physician and Gastroenterologist, Falkirk and District Royal Infirmary, Falkirk

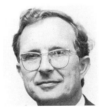

Paul M. Smith MD, MRCP
Consultant Physician, Llandough Hospital, Penarth, South Glamorgan

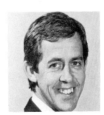

Edwin T. Swarbrick MRCP
Consultant Gastroenterologist, The Wolverhampton Hospitals, West Midlands

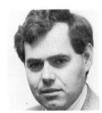

Peter Willoughby MA, MD, MRCP
Consultant Physician and Gastroenterologist, Basildon and Thurrock Health District, Essex

Contents

Preface   ix

1   Doctor, I get heartburn   W.J.S. RUDDELL   1

2   Doctor, my food is sticking   STEPHEN P. KANE   11

3   Doctor, I get terrible indigestion   GRAEME D. KERR   27

4   Doctor, I often feel sick and vomit
EDWIN T. SWARBRICK   41

5   Doctor, I've vomited blood   MICHAEL D. HELLIER   51

6   Doctor, I've always got stomach ache
P.D. FAIRCLOUGH   67

7   Doctor, I've got terrible stomach ache
K.G. BURNAND   77

8   Doctor, I've gone yellow   IAN GILMORE   99

9   Doctor, I've got a big liver   PAUL M. SMITH   115

10   Doctor, my tummy is getting bigger
RUSSELL COWAN   127

11   Doctor, I've got a big spleen   BRIAN GAZZARD   139

12   Doctor, I've suddenly got diarrhoea
MICHAEL GOODMAN   155

13   Doctor, I often get diarrhoea   STUART R. GOULD   171

14   Doctor, I'm allergic to food   V. ALUN JONES AND
      J.O. HUNTER   187

15   Doctor, I've bloody diarrhoea
      PETER WILLOUGHBY   197

16   Doctor, I think I'm anaemic   CHRISTINE LEE   215

17   Doctor, I suffer from terrible wind
      MALCOLM C. BATESON   223

18   Doctor, I'm constipated   JOHN BULL   233

19   Doctor, I think I've got piles   ADAM LEWIS   241

      Index   255

Preface

When a patient consults a doctor about an illness, he complains of symptoms, not of a disease. Most medical books are disease-orientated. *'Doctor, there's something wrong with my guts!'* is different: it is a symptom-orientated guide to gastroenterology. The chapters have all been written by British gastroenterologists and aim to provide a practical guide to the diagnosis, investigation and treatment of patients with gastrointestinal symptoms.

Gastroenterology is mostly an out-patient speciality: only a minority of patients require hospital admission. *'Doctor, there's something wrong with my guts!'* emphasises the type of management that can be undertaken by the general practitioner, rather than elaborate in-patient management.

A recent study of patients referred by general practitioners to a gastroenterology clinic in England revealed that 47.5% of patients had no organic disease. This book reflects the importance of this problem, with four chapters describing the different symptoms which are usually caused by functional bowel disorders — the 'irritable bowel syndrome'. These chapters are sometimes contradictory, but in this they reflect the uncertainties and difficulties associated with the identification and management of these patients. The first step in the management of the irritable bowel syndrome is a confident positive diagnosis, excluding organic disease. All the important organic disorders of the alimentary tract are described in this book, with up-to-date practical advice.

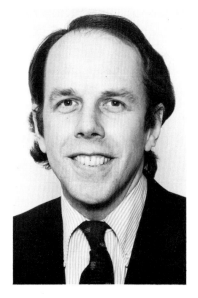

This book has been sponsored by Smith Kline & French Laboratories. Their generosity has allowed an ambitious experiment in medical education, which I hope will be reflected by improved management of our patients with gastrointestinal problems.

ROY POUNDER

Royal Free Hospital, London   July 1983

Acknowledgement for Illustrations

Many of the illustrations for this book have been provided by the authors, but these have been supplemented by pictures kindly provided by a number of other contributors. My particular thanks must go to: Mr Cedric Gilson and Miss Julie Gladwyn (Department of Medical Illustration, Royal Free Hospital), Dr Bob Dick and Dr Les Berger (Department of Radiology, Royal Free Hospital), Professor Kenneth Hobbs (Royal Free Hospital), Dr Andrew Hilson (Department of Medical Physics, Royal Free Hospital), Dr Peter Cotton (Central Middlesex Hospital, London), Dr Paul Brown (Royal Shrewsbury Hospital) and Dr Michael Atkinson (University Hospital, Nottingham).

ALBERTO SANTANA

Royal Free Hospital, London   July 1983

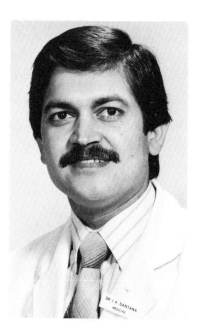

Doctor, I get heartburn

Heartburn is a transient retrosternal or epigastric discomfort usually described as a burning sensation. It may be a sharp or gripping pain and may radiate to the throat, the back and rarely to the arms. It is caused by the effect of refluxing gastric contents onto a sensitive oesophageal mucosa.

Unfortunately it is rare for a patient to cooperate by giving such a clear story. It is even rarer for the patient to add that the pain is associated with acid regurgitation and provoked by stooping or lying flat, and that it hurts to swallow hot or irritant liquids. More commonly the patient may unwittingly add confusion by complaining of 'indigestion', 'dyspepsia' or 'flatulence'. However, the information required to make the diagnosis is almost always available to the astute clinician, and there is no area of medicine where a careful history is more important.

Heartburn is caused by the refluxing of gastric contents onto a sensitive oesophageal mucosa

DIFFERENTIAL DIAGNOSIS

The differential diagnosis of heartburn (Table 1.1) includes many causes of chest and abdominal pain and even a painstaking history will on occasions fail to distinguish heartburn due to gastro-oesophageal reflux from cardiac ischaemia, peptic ulcer, gallstones or the irritable bowel syndrome. Chest pain indistinguishable from *angina* may occur in 10% of patients with oesophagitis, although an association with exertion other than bending is rare. Abnormalities of a resting or exercise ECG may help, but it should be remembered that minor ECG abnormalities may occur during severe oesophageal pain, that oesophageal pain may rarely radiate to the arms, closely simulating angina, and that oesophagitis may coexist with angina.

Peptic ulceration may simulate or coexist with gastro-oesophageal reflux, leading to great difficulty in ascribing all symptoms to a single diagnosis. An episodic history of

Table 1.1 Differential diagnosis in the patient with heartburn

Oesophagitis
Cardiac ischaemia
Peptic ulcer
Gallstones
Irritable bowel syndrome

prominent epigastric pain or vomiting (as opposed to effortless regurgitation) is more characteristic of a peptic ulcer. Marked weight loss suggests the possibility of a *gastric neoplasm*. Rapid worsening of longstanding heartburn may be due to a peptic ulcer or a gastric cancer causing pyloric stenosis. Episodes of severe pain radiating to back or shoulder, associated with bilious vomiting and tenderness in the right hypochondrium, suggest *gallstones*. Most patients with the irritable bowel syndrome or symptomatic *diverticular disease* of the colon will have some abnormality of bowel habit, but the pain can be epigastric.

Most patients with mild symptoms of heartburn can be clearly identified from their history as suffering from gastro-oesophageal reflux and treated accordingly without further investigation.

CLUES FROM THE HISTORY

There are no abnormalities on physical examination that are specific to heartburn so it is fortunate that many clues are available from a well-taken history.

Heartburn is the cardinal system of gastro-oesophageal reflux and is characteristically provoked by:

Heartburn is provoked by bending or stooping, lying flat or large meals

1. Bending or stooping as during housework or gardening.
2. Lying flat, especially in bed at night.
3. Large meals, particularly if greasy.

Gastro-oesophageal reflux occurs painlessly several times a day in healthy individuals, but it rarely causes heartburn. Heartburn occurs when refluxed gastric contents irritate an already inflamed oesophageal mucosa.

Regurgitation is the effortless reflux of gastric contents

Regurgitation of acid or bitter-tasting gastric contents into the mouth is diagnostic of gastro-oesophageal reflux and usually associated with heartburn. The symptom of regurgitation, which is an effortless reflux of gastric contents, must be clearly distinguished from vomiting. Vomiting is a forceful expulsion associated with nausea and abdominal movement; it is not a feature of gastro-oesophageal reflux. Regurgitation is rather like pouring liquid from a jug. The patient will often refer to vomiting when he or she means regurgitation. Recurrent effortless regurgitation of partly digested food during the hour after a meal is characteristic of severe gastro-oesophageal reflux and may be a source of great embarrassment to the patient.

Dysphagia is an abnormal retrosternal sensation or pain occurring within 10 seconds of swallowing. It occurs in two circumstances in the patient with reflux:

1. Hot drinks or irritants, such as alcohol or fruit juice, will commonly provoke acute pain in the patient with an inflamed and sensitive oesophagus due to oesophagitis (Fig. 1.1). This heartburn is usually relieved rapidly by taking an antacid.

2. A peptic oesophageal stricture will eventually cause bolus obstruction which may initially manifest as an episode of severe impact pain, relieved only when the bolus passes through the stricture or is expelled by vomiting. A long history of heartburn followed by slowly-increasing dysphagia to solids and then liquids is usually due to a peptic stricture (see Chapter 2).

<table>
<tr><td>Dysphagia is an abnormal retrosternal sensation or pain occurring with 10 seconds of swallowing</td></tr>
</table>

<table>
<tr><td>A long history of heartburn followed by slowly increasing dysphagia is usually due to peptic stricture</td></tr>
</table>

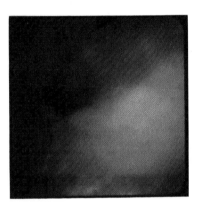

Fig. 1.1   Normal (left) and inflamed (right) gastro-oesophageal mucosa seen at endoscopy.

Dysphagia of this second type is always an indication for *urgent* investigation by barium swallow and subsequent endoscopy and biopsy. Although the absence of previous heartburn and a rapidly progressive history of dysphagia is characteristic of malignancy, particularly in a middle-aged or elderly patient, it must be remembered that malignancy can complicate long-standing gastro-oesophageal reflux, particularly in those patients who have developed columnar metaplasia of the oesophageal mucosa (Barratt's oesophagus). It must never be assumed that dysphagia is due to a benign structure.

PATHOPHYSIOLOGY OF GASTRO-OESOPHAGEAL REFLUX - THE CAUSES OF HEARTBURN

The sensation of heartburn is the end result of many influences on the target organ, the oesophageal mucosa. The sensitivity of the mucosa varies greatly from patient to patient. An understanding of the mechanisms involved may encourage a logical approach to prevention and treatment. The oesophagus may be viewed as the site of a battle between aggressors and defenders, with heartburn the result of victory for the aggressors (Fig. 1.2).

Fig. 1.2   The pathophysiology of gastro-oesophageal reflux.

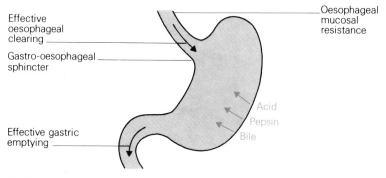

Defence mechanisms

The gastro-oesophageal junction prevents reflux of gastric contents

THE GASTRO-OESOPHAGEAL SPHINCTER. The normal gastro-oesophageal junction has a functional sphincter which prevents reflux of gastric contents, and patients with reflux can be shown by manometry to have lower resting sphincter pressures so that this 'anti-reflux barrier' is more easily breached. There is considerable argument as to whether the presence of a hiatus hernia contributes to sphincter hypotension and the current view is that probably it does not, although it may reduce oesophageal clearing by altering the position of the gastro-oesophageal junction within the chest. The cause of the incompetent sphincter is unknown, although hormonal influences may be important, for example in pregnancy.

OESOPHAGEAL MUCOSAL RESISTANCE. The oesophageal mucosa is damaged by acid, pepsin and bile. However, there is great variation between individuals both in sensitivity to pain and in susceptibility to inflammation and ulceration. The causes of this variation are not known.

The normal oesophagus is cleared by down-going peristaltic waves

OESOPHAGEAL CLEARING. The normal oesophagus is cleared of both swallowed and refluxed material by down-going peristaltic pressure waves. Delayed clearing occurs in patients with oesophagitis, but it is difficult to know which is cause and which is effect. Oesophagitis itself leads to both reduced clearing and a low sphincter pressure. A vicious cycle is thus set up, with reflux oesophagitis leading to poor oesophageal clearing and an incompetent sphincter leading to further reflux (Fig. 1.3). The only way to break the cycle is to heal the oesophagitis.

GASTRIC EMPTYING. Delayed gastric emptying and gastric distension with large volumes increase the frequency and volume of gastro-oesophageal reflux. This is particularly important in patients with pyloric stenosis.

Delayed gastric emptying increases reflux

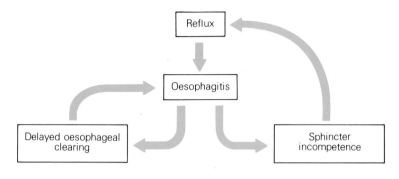

Fig. 1.3 The vicious circle of mechanisms in gastro-oesophageal reflux.

Aggressive factors

Acid, pepsin and bile can all damage the oesophageal mucosa. The damaging effect of bile (alkaline oesophagitis) is particularly important in patients who have had previous gastric surgery which may allow free entry of bile into the stomach, particularly after a gastroenterostomy or Billroth II gastrectomy. Certain tablets, particularly if taken by immobile patients or last thing at night, can cause local damage to the oesophagus (see Chapter 2). It is important that all tablets are washed out of the oesophagus and into the stomach.

Acid, pepsin and bile damage the oesophageal mucosa

INVESTIGATIONS

If the history is typical and not severe, no investigation is required. If there is doubt about the diagnosis, or the symptoms do not respond to simple remedies, further tests are necessary. These may be divided into those which demonstrate reflux, or a potential for reflux, and those which demonstrate mucosal damage (Table 1.2).

To demonstrate reflux

BARIUM SWALLOW. Radiography of the oesophagus should always be accompanied by full examination of stomach and

Table 1.2 Investigations in a patient with heartburn

To demonstrate reflux or potential reflux
Barium swallow
pH monitoring
Oesophageal manometry

To demonstrate mucosal damage
Endoscopy
Mucosal biopsy
Acid perfusion test

duodenum to look for coexisting disease. Unfortunately gastro-oesophageal reflux can be demonstrated in almost all patients by an enthusiastic radiologist, so only the grosser degrees of reflux are significant. Many patients with easily demonstrable reflux have neither oesophagitis nor heartburn. Patients with a sliding hiatus hernia often have some reflux, but the finding of a simple hiatus hernia without oesophagitis is of no significance and should never be accepted as a cause of significant symptoms. A high-quality double-contrast barium swallow may be needed to reveal the effects of reflux: the fine mucosal ulceration of oesophagitis (Fig. 1.4), a discrete oesophageal ulcer (Fig. 1.5) or a benign stricture (Fig. 1.6).

Simple hiatus hernia without oesophagitis is of no clinical significance

---

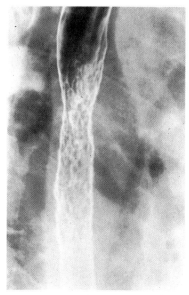

Fig. 1.4 Severe oesophagitis. A double-contrast barium swallow showing fine mucosal ulceration.

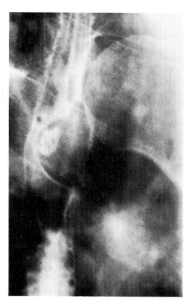

Fig. 1.5 Discrete oesophageal ulcer shown by a barium swallow.

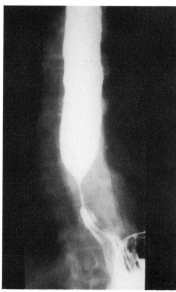

Fig. 1.6 A long fibrous peptic stricture shown by a barium swallow.

OESOPHAGEAL pH MONITORING AND OESOPHAGEAL MANOMETRY. A pH-sensitive electrode placed in the oesophagus can quantify acid reflux. Manometry can be used to measure the sphincter pressure. Both are largely research tools or are used only for difficult clinical problems.

To demonstrate mucosal damage

ENDOSCOPY AND MUCOSAL BIOPSY. Fibreoptic oesophagoscopy and biopsy is the best way to diagnose oesophagitis (Figs 1.7, 1.8). Full inspection of oesophagus, stomach and duodenum is carried out, with target biopsy of any abnormality. Severe oesophagitis is easy to recognise, but the interpretation of less severe inflammation is subject to much observer variation. Combined endoscopy and biopsy is probably the most sensitive and specific test for oesophagitis.

ACID PERFUSION TEST (BERNSTEIN TEST). This is an excellent, simple and much under-used test which can confirm that the patient with 'heartburn' has oesophagitis. A nasogastric tube is passed to the mid oesophagus and is perfused alternately with dilute acid and saline. A positive response, indicating oesophagitis, occurs when the patient's typical 'heartburn' is reproduced by acid and relieved by saline.

MANAGEMENT

Simple changes in lifestyle can pay large dividends for the patient with gastro-oesophageal reflux (Table 1.3). Weight reduction combined with the avoidance of constricting clothing is often all that is necessary to alleviate mild symptoms of heartburn. Patients should avoid large meals and take their evening meal several hours before retiring. Elevation of the bed head on 6 inch (15 cm) blocks is also an effective measure. Foods causing heartburn, such as hot drinks, alcohol or fruit juice, should be avoided. Smoking must be absolutely forbidden as it causes a marked reduction in gastro-oesophageal sphincter pressure. Anticholinergic drugs should be avoided, as they lower sphincter pressure. These simple measures, together with a small dose of antacid taken on

Table 1.3 The therapeutic approach to the patient with heartburn

Phase 1
Lose weight
Stop smoking
Modify diet
Elevate head of bed
Regular antacids

Phase 2
Cimetidine
Metoclopramide or bethanecol
Carbenoxolone/alginate
  (Pyrogastrone)

Phase 3
Anti-reflux surgery

Simple changes in lifestyle pay large dividends for the patient with gastro-oesophageal reflux

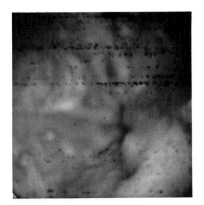 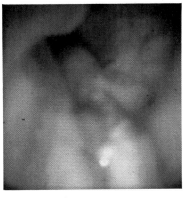

Fig. 1.7 Severe haemorrhagic oesophagitis seen at endoscopy.

Fig. 1.8 Severe oesophagitis with an oesophageal ulcer.

demand, are the only drug therapy required by many patients.

Antacids may be supplemented by preparations containing alginic acid (Gaviscon or Gastrocote) which float on top of the gastric contents. Reflux of this soothing raft may relieve mild oesophagitis.

Patients not improving on these simple measures probably warrant endoscopy and biopsy to confirm the diagnosis of reflux oesophagitis. The next phase of therapy consists of the administration of drugs in addition to previous measures.

Drugs to decrease gastric acidity

H_2-RECEPTOR ANTAGONISTS such as cimetidine and ranitidine are usually effective in relieving heartburn, but there is conflicting evidence about whether they heal oesophagitis. They have no effect on the sphincter and work purely by decreasing acid secretion. The effective dose may be twice that required for duodenal ulcer, for example cimetidine 400 mg qds.

Drugs to reduce reflux

Metoclopramide 10 mg before meals and at night improves gastric enptying and tightens the gastro-oesophageal junction. However, it has not been shown to heal oesophagitis and a careful watch must be kept for extrapyramidal side-effects. Domperidone can be used in the same way, but it has no central nervous system side effects.

Bethanecol is a cholinergic agent which tightens the sphincter and improves oesophageal clearing. Although little used in the United Kingdom it has been shown to heal oesophagitis. The dose is 25 mg before meals and at night, but it may cause mild cholinergic side-effects such as abdominal cramps, urinary frequency and blurred vision.

Drugs to protect the oesophageal mucosa

Carbenoxolone improves gastric mucosal resistance and is available in combination with alginic acid and antacid as Pyrogastrone. A single study showed that one tablet chewed between meals and two at night was effective in healing oesophagitis. Carbenoxolone must be given with care to any elderly patient as it has a potent aldosterone-like activity which may cause severe oedema and hypokalaemia.

A bewildering array of medical treatment for heartburn is available. It is difficult to anticipate which will be helpful for the individual patient. If antacids alone are insufficient, it is reasonable to add cimetidine and either metoclopramide or bethanecol, reserving alginate/carbenoxolone tablets for severe and resistant oesophagitis.

The place of surgery

Surgery should be reserved for those patients who have not responded to an adequate trial of medical therapy. The need for surgery is diminishing as more effective drugs become available. It should be emphasised that the presence of hiatus hernia alone is never an indication for surgery.

Many patients with peptic stricture secondary to oesophagitis can now be managed by repeated endoscopic dilatation without general anaesthesia as an out-patient procedure. Such dilatation should always be accompanied by an intensive medical regimen to heal oesophagitis. Unresponsive severe oesophagitis or a long fibrous stricture may require surgical resection of the stricture and an anti-reflux procedure. The secret is to choose the surgeon for this major procedure carefully: in the right hands the results can be excellent.

The presence of hiatus hernia alone is never an indication for surgery

FURTHER READING

Dodds WJ, Hogan WJ, Helm JF, Dent J (1981) Pathogenesis of reflux oesophagitis. Gastroenterology 81: 376-394.

Leading Article (1982) Gastro-oesophageal reflux in children. Lancet 1: 144-145.

Leading Article (1983) Gastro-oesophageal reflux. Lancet 1: 1081-1082.

Review Article (1981) Tablets and capsules that stick in the oesophagus. Drug Ther Bull 19: 33-34.

Welch CE, Malt RA (1983) Abdominal surgery, part 1. N Engl J Med 308: 624-632.

STEPHEN P. KANE

Doctor, my food is sticking

2

The simple enjoyment of a meal depends not only on the tastes and smells of food and the satisfaction of a replete stomach, but also on the smooth functioning of the voluntary swallowing mechanism, followed by orderly and unobstructed oesophageal peristalsis. These processes are taken for granted until dysfunction or disease leads to an awareness of abnormal swallowing, and the patient presents with the complaint of 'something sticking'. Indeed dysphagia (literally 'difficult eating') is defined in terms of this awareness, which may be painful (odynophagia) or more usually uncomfortable.

Since the lower pharynx and the oesophagus are inaccessible to routine physical examination, a careful history is essential, both to ascertain whether the patient truly has dysphagia and, if he has, to establish provisionally the nature of the lesion, though not necessarily its exact site. It must be emphasised that dysphagia always merits specialist referral and investigation. There is no place for a 'wait and see' policy, unless of course the symptoms are due to something obvious, such as acute tonsillitis.

DIFFFERENTIAL DIAGNOSIS

Whatever its cause, a feeling of mechanical blockage of the oesophagus is a serious symptom, which deserves urgent investigation. Causes of such dysphagia are grouped in Table 2.1, and the following paragraphs highlight the typical symptoms of each group.

Dysphagia always merits specialist referral and investigation

Disorder of pharyngeal musculature and its innervation

Pharyngeal muscle function is impaired in some of the hereditary muscular dystrophies, in dystrophia myotonica and myasthenia gravis, and in the acquired inflammatory disorders, polymyositis and dermatomyositis. The efferent

Table 2.1   The differential diagnosis of dysphagia

Neuromuscular disorders of the pharynx	*Stricturing lesions of the pharynx*	*Stricturing lesions of the oesophagus*
Muscular dystrophies; myasthenia	Mucosal webs	Peptic stricture; erosive oesophagitis
Polymyositis; dermatomyositis	Fibrous strictures	Caustic stricture
Multiple sclerosis	Carcinoma	Post-intubation stricture
Parkinson's disease		Peptic stricture with systemic sclerosis
Brain-stem arterial disease		Carcinoma
		Shatski ring
Motility disorders of the oesophagus	*Extrinsic lesions*	*Sudden onset dysphagia*
Achalasia	Carcinoma of bronchus	Impaction of foreign body
Diffuse spasm	Cervical osteophytes	Impaction of food bolus
Systemic sclerosis	Retrosternal goitre	Candidiasis
	Congenital arterial anomalies	Mediastinal radiotherapy
	Atheromatous aorta	Drug-induced oesophageal ulcer
	Giant left atrium	Intramural oesophageal haematoma

nerves may be damaged in poliomyelitis, Guillain-Barré polyneuritis and motor neuron disease. Brain-stem lesions which result in dysphagia include demyelinating plaques of multiple sclerosis, thrombotic and embolic occlusions of the brain-stem arteries, and the pseudobulbar palsy which follows bilateral middle cerebral artery occlusion. Extrapyramidal syndromes, particularly Parkinson's disease, may also cause dysphagia.

Neuromuscular pharyngeal disorders lead to difficulties with the initiation of swallowing both solids and liquids, a problem which becomes exaggerated when the patient is embarrassed or stressed. After several abortive attempts, a successful swallow may be accompanied by immediate regurgitation of fluid via the nose or coughing, due to failure of closure of the nasopharynx or the larynx, respectively.

Neuromuscular disorders lead to difficulty with the initiation of swallowing

Stricturing lesions of the pharynx

Patients with lesions in this site are uncommon, representing a small proportion of all patients with dysphagia. They include those with carcinomas of the hypopharynx and cervical oesophagus, and patients with benign mucosal webs and short submucosal fibrous strictures. The pharyngeal web, which accompanies chronic iron-deficiency anaemia (Plummer-Vinson syndrome) and reputedly disappears on repletion of iron stores, is now rare, although its malignant potential is recognised.

Lesions which constrict the pharynx cause a sensation of food sticking at the moment of swallowing, often accompanied by the prompt return of the food bolus to the mouth. With worsening constriction, liquids have to be sipped rather than gulped.

Malignant pharyngeal lesions will generally present with a short history of worsening symptoms. Benign lesions such as webs have a longer history, often with intermittent symptoms.

Stricturing lesions of the oesophagus

Benign and malignant strictures of the oesophagus are by far the commonest group of disorders presenting to the gastroesterologist as dysphagia.

Benign and malignant strictures of the oesophagus are by far the most common causes of dysphagia

The benign 'peptic' stricture arising near the gastro-oesophageal junction is particularly common. The patient is usually middle-aged or elderly, often female and often taking a non-steroidal anti-inflammatory drug for arthritis. Such a patient usually gives a long history of reflux symptoms. Some patients with reflux may complain of painful dysphagia in association with lower oesophageal erosions and ulceration, yet significant stricturing cannot be demonstrated either radiologically or endoscopically (Fig. 2.1).

Apart from ulceration and scarring due to gastro-oesophageal reflux of acid, pepsin or bile, lower oesophageal strictures may also follow mucosal damage due to the ingestion of corrosive substances (e.g. Lysol) taken accidentally or with suicidal intent. The reflux associated with a prolonged period of nasogastric intubation can produce a stricture due to localised oesophageal damage. Peptic strictures are a common complication of the free gastro-oesophageal reflux which accompanies involvement of the lower oesophageal musculature by systemic sclerosis.

The second most common cause of an oesophageal stricture is carcinoma of the thoracic oesophagus, which reaches its peak incidence in patients in their sixties. Most tumours are squamous carcinomas. A small proportion are adeno-carcinomata either arising in metaplastic gastric epithelium in the lower oesophagus (Barrett's oesophagus) or originating within the gastric fundus and invading the mucosa or sub-mucosa of the distal oesophagus. The five-year survival figure is 5% or less and oesophageal cancer kills 3,500 people annually in England and Wales.

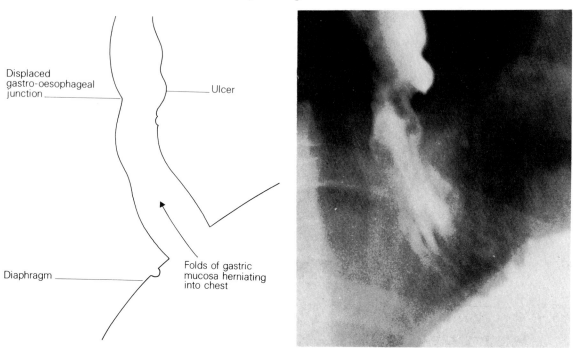

Displaced gastro-oesophageal junction

Ulcer

Diaphragm

Folds of gastric mucosa herniating into chest

Fig. 2.1 Oesophageal ulcer above a hiatus hernia in a patient presenting with intermittent dysphagia and some heartburn.

Whether the stricture is benign or malignant, the patient will complain of a sensation of food sticking, which occurs several seconds after swallowing. He may localise the sticking sensation to a point or area anywhere from the hyoid bone to the epigastrium: but his localisation bears no relationship to the true site of the lesion and it should be disregarded. Only the time interval from 'swallowing' to 'sticking' gives a clue as to how far below the pharynx the lesion is likely to be found. Sticking occurs initially with bulky solids such as steak, dry bread and roast potatoes, whereas liquids can be swallowed fast without discomfort. This lack of dysphagia for liquids, in all but pin-hole benign strictures and advanced malignant strictures, helps to distinguish mechanical lesions from motility disorders of the oesophagus.

Benign strictures usually cause a slow evolution of symptoms

Patients with benign peptic strictures usually experience a slow evolution of their symptoms, and may have experienced intermittent dysphagia for solids a year or more before presenting to their doctor. On some days they may still be able to eat soft foods without experiencing a sensation of sticking. Associated oesophagitis will frequently have caused pain after hot drinks or alcoholic spirits have been swallowed. Patients may have lost weight, but frequently they maintain their calorie and nutrient intake despite adjusting to a more sloppy or liquid diet.

In contrast, patients with malignant strictures present with a history of weeks, rather than months, of dysphagia. From the first meal which caused dysphagia, solids will stick on almost all subsequent occasions. Initially patients may also feel impact pain, but this lessens while dysphagia relentlessly worsens. The patient may continue to feel hungry, but he learns to eat little and rapidly loses weight.

One other less common obstructing lesion of the lower oesophagus merits brief consideration, the Schatski ring (Fig. 2.2). It is usually found immediately above a hiatus hernia, and consists of an upper layer of oesophageal mucosa and a lower layer of gastric mucosa, separated by lamina propria and some smooth muscle. Such rings may be asymptomatic or may cause intermittent, but sudden and total, obstruction due to impaction of a bolus of solid food.

> Malignant strictures present with a history of weeks of dysphagia, rather than months

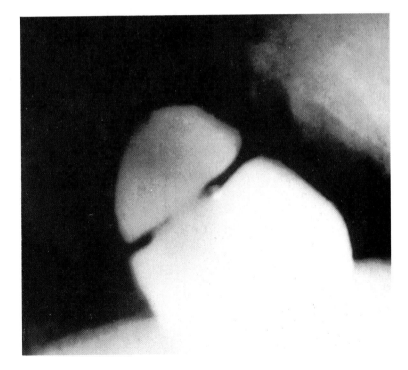

Fig. 2.2   A Shatski ring above a small hiatus hernia.

Motility disorders of the oesophagus

The two main disorders are achalasia and diffuse oesophageal spasm, but both are very uncommon.

The primary abnormality in achalasia is degeneration of Auerbach's plexus, the post-ganglionic nerve fibres which supply oesophageal smooth muscle. Except in the case of Chagas' disease, where this degenerative process is known to follow trypanosomal infection, the aetiology of achalasia remains unknown. It can start at any age. The lack of neural control of the smooth muscle results in a loss of the primary peristaltic wave which normally empties the oesophagus of each food or fluid bolus. Moreover, the lower oesophageal sphincter, which would normally relax as the bolus is propelled towards it, fails to do so. The oesophagus gradually dilates to become a flaccid bag containing up to 200 ml of saliva, fluid and food debris. The oesophageal contents pass with difficulty through the high pressure zone of the lower oesophageal sphincter, but they may also be regurgitated into the mouth or aspirated into the trachea, particularly when the patient lies down at night. Achalasia may also cause spasms of retrosternal pain.

In the rarer syndrome of diffuse oesophageal spasm (Fig. 2.3), gross muscular hypertrophy is the main pathological finding, while pre- and post-ganglionic neuronal degeneration is inconstant. Segmenting, non-propulsive high pressure contractions develop in the lower oesophagus, and a high pressure is usually maintained in the lower oesophageal sphincter. Marked radiological and manometric abnormalities may be found in asymptomatic subjects, while in others comparable changes are associated with oesophageal colic, often waking the patient at night and simulating the pain of myocardial infarction.

Both disorders are characterised by dysphagia which is experienced seconds after completion of the voluntary swallow, but which is similar for solids and liquids. Symptoms are worse if the patient tries to eat and drink fast. If a meal is taken slowly it can usually be finished and substantial weight loss is unusual. In diffuse spasm, dysphagia may be episodic, and sometimes provoked by cold drinks.

In systemic sclerosis aperistalsis of the lower oesophagus causes mild dysphagia which becomes severe only when incompetence of the lower sphincter leads to oesophagitis and stricturing.

In achalasia the oesophagus gradually dilates to become a flaccid bag

Fig. 2.3   Diffuse oesophageal spasm. The barium meal shows segmentation in association with marked tertiary contractions.

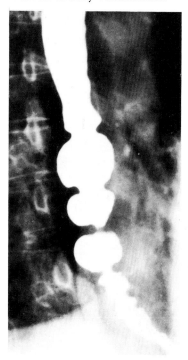

Pharyngeal pouches

A pharyngeal pouch may cause intermittent dysphagia, the patient describing immediate return of food or liquid to the mouth on swallowing. Some regurgitation may occur hours after a meal, particularly when the patient is recumbent. A specific feature of this disorder is that, when drinking, the patient may become aware of a soft gurgling swelling appearing in the neck.

Extrinsic lesions

The site of compression will determine the timing of the patient's awareness of food sticking in relation to swallowing.

Carcinoma of the bronchus is the commonest malignancy in the United Kingdom. It may on occasions present with dysphagia, due either to local spread of the tumour around or into the oesophageal wall or to compression of the oesophagus by nodal metastases (Fig. 2.4).

Carcinoma of the bronchus may present with dysphagia

Large anterior osteophytes, associated with severe cervical spondylosis, occasionally indent the cervical oesophagus to produce some dysphagia. More rarely, a retropharyngeal abscess will cause the acute onset of difficulty with swallowing.

Within the thorax the oesophagus may be compressed by a large retrosternal goitre, by congenitally anomalous branches of the aorta, or more commonly by an unfolded atheromatous aortic arch. The large left atrium typical of mitral stenosis can frequently be shown radiologically to narrow the lumen of the lower oesophagus, but it is exceptional for this to be associated with significant symptoms.

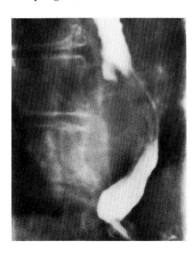

Fig. 2.4   Carcinoma of the bronchus invading the oesophagus.

Sudden onset dysphagia

Acute and complete dysphagia results from the oesophageal impaction of a foreign body or a large bolus of poorly chewed food, which is more likely to happen if there is already an oesophageal abnormality, such as a stricture or a diverticulum.

Symptomatic oesophageal candidiasis almost always arises in debilitated patients, paticularly those receiving broad-spectrum antibiotics, corticosteroids or cytotoxic drugs or with advanced malignant disease. It is easy to overlook the patient's complaint of painful dysphagia when he or she is already anorexic. An additional clue will be the complaint of a sore dry mouth due to associated oral candidiasis.

Patients who are in the midst of, or who have recently completed, a course of radiotherapy to the mediastinum may complain of dysphagia.

Iatrogenic oesophageal ulceration can present dramatically with chest pain, which is worsened by attempts to swallow solids or liquids. A variety of tablets and capsules, particularly if taken without a drink and just before going to bed, will stick in the oesophagus and cause ulceration which is worsened by the adherence of subsequent tablets. The anticholinergic drug emepronium bromide, and both oxytetracycline and doxycycline, have been particularly implicated in causing this syndrome, although other culprits include aspirin and slow-release potassium. When the offending drug is stopped, mediastinal pain and odynophagia generally disappear within a few days, though occasionally oesophageal stricturing follows.

Pseudodysphagias

The patient presents with the complaint that his food 'sticks', that there is a feeling of 'something stuck' or that he 'cannot swallow his food'. Further questioning reveals that these symptoms do not occur either during the voluntary act of swallowing or during the few seconds immediately following it which represent the normal time of involuntary transit of a bolus to the stomach.

The patient may be describing 'cortical inhibition', a failure to initiate the swallowing of chewed food, which is retained in the mouth and eventually spat out. This can be a feature of the anorexia which accompanies many illnesses, particularly malignant disease, of dementia or of severe depression. This symptom merits consideration in its own right, but should not prompt needless searches for an oesophageal abnormality.

Similarly, the patient whose 'stuck' feeling turns out to be a sensation of tightness or lumpiness in the throat, either acute or chronic, which actually diminishes on swallowing, is almost certainly describing a symptom of anxiety. Here, the GP, far from referring the patient to his ENT or gastroenterologist collegue, is in the best position to explore his patient's psyche. However, the patient who relates a feeling like a crumb stuck in his throat, which he cannot clear, does merit an ENT opinion, for he could have an early pharyngeal tumour.

Finally there is the patient who points to his epigastrium and says 'my food seems to stick here', but who on further enquiry reveals that, while solids and liquids go down satisfactorily, feelings of upper abdominal fullness and discomfort develop either while eating or within a few minutes of completing a meal. If symptoms develop while eating, the patient may well start to restrict his food intake. Resulting weight loss suggests that the possibility of a gastric carcinoma must be explored. Similar symptoms are, of course, common after previous partial or total gastrectomy. Lesser degrees of postprandial fullness may be due to a gastric motility disorder or, like cortical inhibition, may be the patient's way of expressing anorexia. A barium meal examination or an endoscopy is fully justifiable in the investigation of a patient presenting with this type of pseudodysphagia, but attention should not be focussed on the oesophagus.

ABNORMALITIES ON EXAMINATION

A careful physical examination of the mouth, neck, chest and abdomen is essential in any patient presenting with swallowing difficulties, and a neurological examination is also vital when the patient's symptoms suggest pharyngeal incoordination (for example, liquids regurgitating down the nose).

However, the majority of patients with dysphagia have few if any helpful physical signs. General evidence of recent weight loss suggests carcinoma, and signs such as pallor, clubbing or jaundice may give useful leads. Abnormalities to be sought in the mouth are patches of *Candida* infection (Fig. 2.5), acute

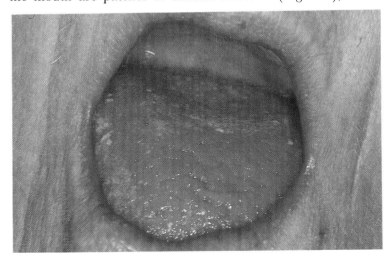

Fig. 2.5   Candidal infection of the mouth.

tonsillitis, oropharyngeal ulceration or tumour, and the wasted fasciculating tongue of motor neuron disease. The patient may have an obvious dysarthria of a pseudobulbar or parkinsonian type; a parkinsonian or myopathic facies should be noted. Clues in the neck may include a palpable pharyngeal pouch, a large goitre or enlarged lymph nodes due to metastatic spread from pharyngeal, oesophageal, gastric or bronchial carcinoma.

In the chest, the examiner might find evidence of bronchial carcinoma such as lobar collapse or pleural effusion, or possibly the physical signs of mitral stenosis. In the abdomen, the presence of an epigastric mass suggests gastric carcinoma as the source of the patient's symptoms. An enlarged hard irregular liver raises the likelihood of secondaries from a malignant tumour of the oesophagus, bronchus or stomach.

INVESTIGATIONS

Haematology and biochemistry

The extent to which both routine and more specialised haematological and biochemical tests should be employed in managing the patient presenting with difficulty in swallowing must depend upon the working diagnosis. For example, both peptic strictures and carcinoma of the oesophagus are frequently accompanied by iron-deficiency anaemia. A fall in the serum albumin may result from malnutrition in a patient with advanced carcinoma of the oesophagus. In the same disease a rising hepatic alkaline phosphatase suggests liver metastases and should prompt an hepatic scintiscan or ultrasound, if only to spare the patient a needless attempted resection.

Radiology

In the routine investigation of dysphagia, the anatomy and pathophysiology of the pharynx, oesophagus and upper stomach should be examined by a careful barium swallow. This test should if possible precede oesophagoscopy, even though a direct look at the oesophageal mucosa is going to be necessary in the common disorders presenting with dysphagia, peptic stricture and oesophageal cancer.

Radiology and endoscopy should be regarded as complementary: the first shows in longitudinal section both the

Barium swallow should precede oesophagoscopy

static contours of the upper food passages and the dynamic way in which liquid barium or a solid barium-soaked bolus of bread is handled. It can show the level of a stricture without the hazard of perforation. The second looks in greater detail, but in transverse section, at the oesophageal and gastric mucosa, and provides opportunities both for biopsy and for therapy. It gives little opportunity, however, for assessing disordered physiology, and the endoscopist can all too easily make the error of assuming that, because the mucosa looks normal, there can be nothing wrong with the oesophagus.

The radiologist may confirm the aspiration and nasal regurgitation of fluid characteristic of neuromuscular disorders of the pharynx, or he may observe the atonic dilated oesophagus of achalasia (Fig. 2.6) with the 'beaked' lower end due to a non-relaxing lower oesophageal sphincter. Similarly he may show the 'corkscrew' oesophagus, with its marked tertiary contractions, typical of the diffuse spasm. Radiological examination should also demonstrate pouches, diverticula, webs, rings and strictures, both benign and malignant. Typically, the benign peptic stricture is found in the lower oesophagus above a hiatus hernia. It is short and centrally placed, and the luminal silhouette both above and below the stricture is convex (Figs 2.7, 2.8). Carcinomatous strictures, though most common in the lower third of the oesophagus, can

Fig. 2.6 Achalasia. The moderately dilated oesophagus of a 20-year-old patient presenting with a year's history of dysphagia for solids and liquids, with spontaneous chest pain.

Fig. 2.7 A short peptic stricture above a large hiatus hernia in an elderly lady with a 15-year history of heartburn and a 10-year history of dysphagia for solids. After one dilatation she was able to change her diet from 'Complan' to fillet steak!

Fig. 2.8 Peptic stricture in an 82-year-old woman who had taken non-steroidal anti-inflammatory drugs for many years for severe osteoarthritis of the hip. These had probably contributed to her oesophageal ulceration and stricture.

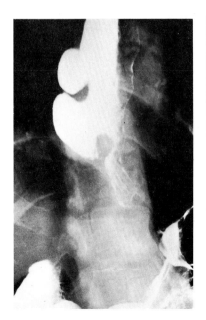

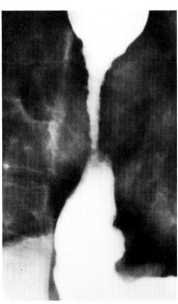

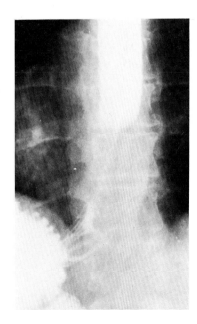

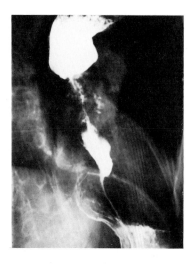

Fig. 2.9 Barium swallow of a 48-year-old patient with a two-month history of progressive dysphagia for solids and later for liquids too. The shouldering at both ends of the stricture is typical of carcinoma.

also occur in the middle or upper thirds. In contrast to benign strictures they are long, eccentrically placed and irregular and their silhouette is shouldered (Fig. 2.9).

Radiology should also help to pinpoint extrinsic compression of the pharynx or oesophagus by osteophytes, major arteries, tumours or a large left atrium. A request for a barium swallow examination should always be accompanied by a request for postero-anterior and lateral chest radiographs so that conditions such as bronchial carcinoma are not missed.

Endoscopy

Endoscopy and mucosal biopsy are mandatory if a stricture is seen on X-ray. It is not usually a problem for the endoscopist to distinguish peptic from carcinomatous strictures. The former almost always have longitudinal streaks of erosive oesophagitis extending for up to 10 cm above them. The stricture itself, though often too narrow to admit even an 8 mm gastroscope, is situated centrally, and is round and superficially ulcerated (Fig. 2.10). If an endoscope can be passed through it either before or after dilatation, normal gastric mucosa will be found immediately below it, usually lining a hiatus hernia. A malignant stricture, on the other hand, does not generally have any oesophagitis above it. The oesophageal mucosa becomes abruptly irregular, lumpy and ulcerated, narrowing the lumen over a variable length. Most or all of the circumference is involved, but the bulk of the tumour may be on one side so that the lumen becomes eccentric (Fig. 2.11). Biopsies and brushings for cytology must be taken from all oesophageal strictures to exclude malignancy.

Endoscopy is also of considerable value in the diagnosis of oesophageal moniliasis or drug-induced oesophageal ulceration, and in establishing the presence of severe reflux oesophagitis in the absence of a stricture. All these lesions may go undetected by contrast radiological examination.

Oesophageal manometry

Oesophageal manometry is available only in some specialised centres. It has considerably advanced our understanding of normal and abnormal oesophageal motor function, and has proved particularly valuable in showing the disorders of peristalsis and of lower oesophageal sphincter function that characterise achalasia and diffuse spasm. If there remains doubt as to whether or not a patient suffers from one of these conditions, then it is worth considering referral to a unit where manometry is carried out.

MANAGEMENT

This section will deal mainly with the treatment of peptic strictures, oesophageal carcinoma and achalasia. However, brief mention should be made of the management of neuromuscular problems in the pharynx. Some patients who cannot swallow either solids or liquids seem to cope better with a semi-liquid diet. If even this causes choking, then nasogastric intubation with a fine-bore feeding tube should be considered as a short- or long-term measure. This is justified even in patients with motor neuron disease, if dysphagia and malnutrition overshadow other neurological disabilities.

Peptic strictures

Peptic strictures, once established, are best treated by some form of dilatation, although in younger fitter patients the possibility of surgical repair of the associated hiatus hernia or even resection of the stricture should be considered. However, most patients are elderly, with far greater risks from major surgery than from repeated dilatations.

Dilatation is usually carried out with the Eder-Peustow technique. Under sedation, the stricture is visualised with a fibreoptic endoscope, a guide-wire is passed through the narrowed lumen into the stomach and the endoscope is withdrawn. A series of metal olives of increasing size are then threaded along the guide-wire and are gently moved back and forth through the stricture. The risk of oesophageal perforation is small, and patients can be discharged home on the day of the procedure or after an overnight stay. Dilatation may have to be repeated on one or more occasions over subsequent months or years, though the need for further dilatation decreases with time.

The patient should be advised on measures to reduce gastro-oesophageal reflux (see Chapter 1), and any ulcerogenic drugs should if possible be withdrawn. Continuous maintenance treatment with cimetidine 400 mg nocte decreases the need for repeated dilatations. Larger doses of an H_2-receptor antagonist may be needed, but even as long-term treatment this may be an acceptable alternative to major surgery.

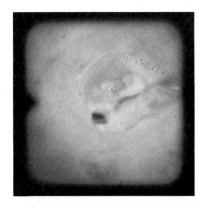

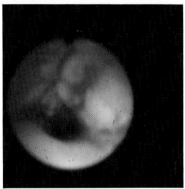

Fig. 2.10 A peptic stricture seen at endoscopy.

Fig. 2.11 Oesophageal carcinoma seen at endoscopy.

Oesophageal carcinoma

Oesophageal carcinoma is usually inoperable at the time of presentation, by virtue of extensive local spread, lymph node involvement or distant metastases. The patient is often elderly, malnourished and suffers from coexistent cardiac or respiratory disease. Nonetheless, resection offers the only prospect of cure and should be considered in younger patients without such complications. Local spread may be difficult to assess preoperatively, but computerised axial tomography may in future provide an early guide to operability.

For the patient with an inoperable tumour, adequate palliation is essential, since the alternative is starvation due to progressive dysphagia, and a stage when even saliva can not be swallowed. Radiotherapy is a well-established treatment which provides considerable though temporary, symptomatic relief for many patients with squamous tumours, though adenocarcinomas are usually radio-resistant. As an alternative, the palliative intubation of oesophageal and high gastric cancers has long been used, though formerly this required a laparotomy. However, a variety of prosthetic tubes are now available which can be introduced through a malignant stricture along an endoscopically positioned guide-wire, the stricture having first been dilated. Though there is an 8-9% risk of oesophageal perforation, and a significant mortality (about 4%), this is lower than the immediate mortality associated with surgical placement of prostheses. Obstruction and tube migration can follow either approach, but if the tube remains patent and in position, dysphagia may be relieved for weeks or months.

Achalasia

Achalasia has traditionally been treated either by pneumatic dilatation of the lower oesophageal sphincter or by Heller's cardiomyotomy. Both approaches aim to weaken the sphincter rather than to destroy it, since an incompetent sphincter will lead to gastro-oesophageal reflux, made worse by the inability of the lower oesophagus to clear gastric contents by peristalsis. Both dilatation and surgery produce long-term symptomatic relief in 70-90% of patients, though repeated dilatations are required over the years in some cases. Both forms of treatment have been tried in diffuse spasm, but with only limited success.

FURTHER READING

Edwards DAW (1976) Discriminatory value of symptoms in the differential diagnosis of dysphagia. Clin Gastroenterol 5 : 49-57.

Edwards DAW (1980) Concepts of oesophageal disorders. J R Soc Med 73: 402-404.

Ogilvie AL, Fergerson R, Atkinson M (1980) Outlook with conservative treatment of peptic oesophageal stricture. Gut 21 : 23-25.

GRAEME D. KERR

Doctor, I get terrible indigestion

3

'Indigestion' is a term usually used by patients to describe symptoms related to the upper abdomen and chest, but at times even referring to lower abdominal discomfort and disturbances of bowel function. To complicate matters further, 'indigestion' not only means different things to different patients but may also be used to describe different symptoms in the same patient at different times!

Indigestion means different things to different patients

DIFFERENTIAL DIAGNOSIS

The differential diagnosis for indigestion (Table 3.1) is extremely wide, involving diseases not only of the stomach and duodenum, but also the whole range of the organs sited in the middle part of the body. This range of diagnoses provides a considerable diagnostic challange, hence serious indigestion almost invariably demands hospital investigation.

CLUES FROM THE HISTORY

The patient uses 'indigestion' as a form of medical jargon, but the doctor must identify the exact symptoms which are obscured by this term. Leading questions are often required to elicit the complaint that troubles the patient. Table 3.2 lists the different groups of symptoms that may be covered by the patient's complaint of simple indigestion. Even when a precise history has been obtained, the exact clinical diagnosis is often difficult, even for a most experienced physician. Symptoms such as pain, weight loss, nocturnal waking or relief or aggravation by eating often fail to discriminate between the different diagnoses. The combinations and permutations of different symptom patterns are so wide that an appropriately programmed computer may, in the future, sort out a more accurate differential diagnosis than an experienced doctor.

Table 3.1 Diseases causing 'indigestion'

Ischaemic heart disease
Oesophageal reflux
Duodenal ulcer
Gastric ulcer
Gastric carcinoma
Symptomatic cholelithiasis
Chronic pancreatitis
Bowel disorders:
   irritable bowel disease
   carcinoma of transverse colon
   vascular insufficiency
Alcohol-induced symptoms
Non-organic disorders

Table 3.2 Complaints the patient may describe as 'indigestion'

Angina of effort
Upper abdominal pain
Flatulence
Abdominal distension
Nausea and anorexia
Nausea with vomiting
Heartburn
Dysphagia

Ischaemic heart diseases

A diagnosis of ischaemic heart disease may be indicated by retrosternal or high epigastric pain clearly related to effort, and radiating to typical sites such as the neck, jaw, shoulder and arm. Symptoms are clearly relieved by rest but recur under similar circumstances, and are relieved by glyceryl trinitrate.

Heartburn

Heartburn is the classical symptom of gastro-oesophageal reflux. Oesophageal reflux is a normal physiological event but it gives rise to symptoms when the oesophageal mucosa is inflamed. Many patients have a hiatal hernia without significant symptoms of reflux.

Flatulence

Belching is the regurgitation of air swallowed during eating, drinking or at other times. If unaccompanied by heartburn or other dyspeptic symptoms, it is usually not associated with serious disease and it may reflect an anxiety state.

Duodenal ulcer

Patients have a high probability of duodenal ulcer if they describe intermittent symptoms of epigastric pain which they can locate by finger point; pain which is worse before meals and relieved by taking food or antacids; or epigastric pain which wakes the patient at night, commonly at about 2 a.m., when it is again relieved by food or antacids.

The diagnosis is further strengthened if the history is clearly episodic with symptoms present for a few months at a time, followed by periods of remission. A history of prompt and complete symptomatic relief by an earlier course of an H_2-receptor antagonist suggests an acid-related illness. A strong family history of peptic ulceration in a male patient further strengthens the diagnosis. There may be associated symptoms of heartburn and occasional vomiting.

Gastric ulcer

It is usually not possible to differentiate between gastric and duodenal ulceration by symptoms alone. Gastric ulcer occurs more commonly in females than does duodenal ulcer and the patients are often older, over the age of 40. Pain relief associated with food may be short-lived and thus the patient may believe that food aggravates the pain. Anorexia, nausea and weight loss are more prominent symptoms of gastric ulcer than of duodenal ulcer.

Gastric cancer

A brief history of dyspepsia occurring in a patient over the age of 55 should raise the strong suspicion of gastric cancer. When symptoms of daily pain, discomfort and early repletion are added, the probability of gastric cancer becomes high. Weight loss, anorexia and nausea are common symptoms of advanced malignancy.

A short history of dyspepsia with daily pain and early repletion suggest gastric cancer

Symptomatic cholelithiasis

Clear-cut, well remembered attacks of pain, usually of sudden onset, sited in the epigastrium or below the right costal margin, passing through to the back on the right, and of variable intensity from mild to severely incapacitating, are typical of cholelithiasis. The pain is produced by stones impacting in the cystic duct or the common bile duct. In this latter instance there may be associated features of intermittent jaundice, dark urine and pale stools, or even episodic fever and rigors associated with infection in the biliary tree. Symptoms of gallbladder disease may be precipitated by the ingestion of fatty foods, but this is by no means a universal or specific event.

Sudden episodes of clear-cut epigastric pain are typical of cholelithiasis

Gallstones are often present without symptoms. They may be found in close association with other diseases, such as diverticular disease of the colon or irritable bowel, a peptic ulcer or oesophageal reflux. Surgical relief of cholelithiasis may leave such a patient continuing to suffer symptoms from other causes.

Chronic pancreatitis

This less common condition may be associated with chronic alcohol abuse or cholelithiasis. It presents as deep boring upper abdominal discomfort, radiating to the back. There may be other symptoms of pancreatic insufficiency - steatorrhoea and possibly diabetes mellitus. Similar symptoms of shorter duration may be associated with carcinoma of the pancreas,

Carcinoma of the pancreas is notorious for its late presentation but this condition is notorious for its late presentation, when the patient is cachectic and jaundiced.

Bowel disorders

Symptoms of abdominal pain occurring soon after eating, in a patient with vascular disease elsewhere, may indicate vascular insufficiency of the gut.

Carcinoma, particularly in the transverse colon, may give symptoms confused with 'indigestion'. Patients present with vague diffuse abdominal pain which they cannot clearly locate or describe. Bowel habit may not be disturbed. A pain or discomfort that tends to be felt diffusely over the abdomen, or in varying sites, and which is associated with abdominal bloating and flatulence, is usually not organic and may represent an irritable bowel syndrome. It may be associated with bowel disturbances and the passage of small stools like rabbit droppings, constipation or variable diarrhoea. It should be stressed, however, that in many instances these symptoms warrant investigation before the final diagnosis of irritable bowel syndrome is made.

Alcohol-induced dyspepsia

High alcohol ingestion, which may be social or addictive, may induce symptoms of dyspepsia, particularly morning nausea and retching. Alcohol abuse should be suspected in patients with such symptoms who are also smokers and who often have social problems such as marital disharmony. Alcohol-induced disease is an increasing social disability not confined to men.

Non-organic dyspepsia

Non-organic dyspepsia may account for as many as 40-50% of problems referred to a hospital gastrointestinal clinic. The majority of these patients are suffering from the irritable bowel syndrome.

ABNORMALITIES ON EXAMINATION

In many instances physical examination of the dyspeptic patient may not reveal any clinical abnormality. The clinician should take account of the signs listed in Table 3.3.

Table 3.3   Specific signs in indigestion

General examination
General well-being
Evidence of weight loss
Anaemia
Condition of peripheral
   vasculature
Cardiac state
Oedema

Abdominal examination
Tenderness
Abdominal masses
Hepatosplenomegaly
Ascites
Rectal examination

The presence of a gastric succussion splash indicates pyloric obstruction which may be caused by stenosis following duodenal ulceration or a pyloric malignancy. There may be no relevant finding in patients with symptoms of oesophageal reflux or with duodenal or gastric ulcer. Gastric or bowel malignancy may present as a palpable mass and may be associated with anaemia. The presence of hepatic enlargement, with possible irregularity of the liver surface, may indicate hepatic secondaries. Lymph gland enlargement should not be overlooked, particularly in the left supraclavicular fossa, as this may also indicate spread from a gastric carcinoma (Fig. 3.1). Rectal examination may reveal pelvic secondaries seeding from a gastric carcinoma.

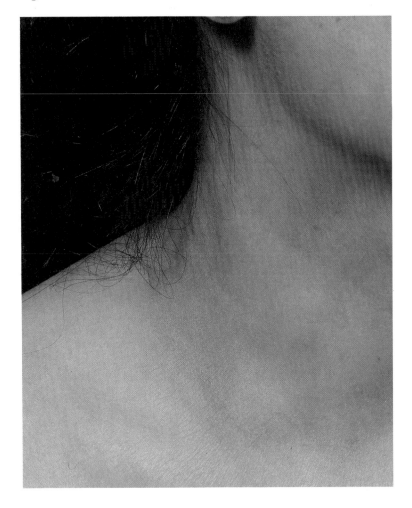

Fig. 3.1 Lymph node metastases from carcinoma of the stomach.

INVESTIGATIONS

Laboratory

The *blood count* may show evidence of iron deficiency anaemia, indicating an ulcerative lesion in the gastrointestinal tract. An increase in mean corpuscular volume (MCV) may be associated with alcohol abuse. Anaemia, associated with an elevated platelet count or ESR, raises the suspicion of malignancy.

Liver function tests may show evidence of an elevated alkaline phosphatase. A gamma glutamyl transferase estimation would indicate that this was of hepatic and not bony origin. Elevated alkaline phosphatase may be associated with biliary tract disease, hepatic malignancy, either primary or secondary, and alcohol abuse.

Urea and electrolyte estimations should be performed in patients with persistent vomiting. Uraemia may present with dyspepsia and vomiting. Hypercalcaemia, usually due to hyperparathyroidism, is a cause of nausea and it may be associated with duodenal ulcer. Serum amylase levels are usually not helpful in chronic pancreatitis except following an acute exacerbation.

Radiology

A *chest X-ray* may be helpful in eliminating other diseases and may also demonstrate an incarcerated hiatal hernia.

Plain X-ray of the abdomen should be considered as it may provide helpful information in demonstrating gallstones or pancreatic calcification, indicating chronic pancreatitis. Fluid levels may be revealed in the bowel, indicating bowel obstruction. A dilated stomach containing a granular mass of old food may be seen in pyloric stenosis.

BARIUM MEAL. Although endoscopy has become the major means of examination of the upper gastrointestinal tract, a barium meal can still produce useful information. Motility disorders of the oesophagus may be best demonstrated by this means; the presence of oesophageal reflux is better assessed radiologically than by endoscopy; and hiatal hernia is more easily defined by this technique.

A barium meal may show gastric lesions like gastric ulcer or carcinoma. It can demonstrate the presence of a duodenal ulcer. However, after gastric surgery, such as vagotomy and pyloroplasty or partial gastrectomy, ulceration is reported less reliably, owing to the distortion inevitably produced by the surgical procedure.

Gastric emptying and the presence of partial pyloric obstruction are better assessed radiologically than by endoscopy.

The barium meal examination will also examine the duodenal loop and the upper loops of the jejunum and may reveal an abnormality in the region of the head of the pancreas, e.g. pancreatic carcinoma (Fig. 3.2), or other lesions such as duodenal and jejunal diverticula.

The following radiological findings may lead to a request for an endoscopic examination:

1. A negative examination in the presence of positive symptoms.

2. Suspected mucosal lesions, not defined on radiology.

3. Gastric ulceration.

4. Oesophageal or gastric tumour.

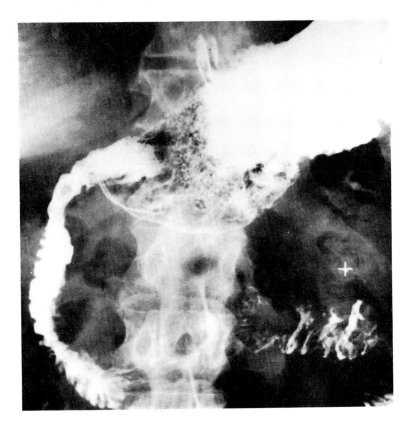

Fig. 3.2 Carcinoma of the pancreas causing a 'reversed three' sign in the duodenal loop.

ORAL CHOLECYSTOGRAM. In patients with upper abdominal pain suggestive of biliary tract disease, an oral cholecystogram may be the first examination requested. It may demonstrate the presence of gallstones or a non-functioning gallbladder. The non-opacification of the gallbladder usually indicates disease, but one must be sure that the patient has taken the contrast agent. Liver disease may prevent adequate excretion of the contrast agent. When investigating dyspepsia some hospital departments will perform a barium meal and oral cholecystogram at the same visit, as it is often difficult to be sure which of the two is the more appropriate primary investigation.

ULTRASOUND EXAMINATION. This technique for the investigation of the upper abdomen, and more specifically the gallbladder and biliary tree, is rapidly replacing oral cholecystography as a primary investigation. It is a non-invasive examination and may show the presence of gallstones (Fig. 3.3) or a dilated biliary tree. It also has the advantage of being able to show abnormalities of associated structures such as hepatic lesions, major lesions of the pancreas and lesions of adjacent structures such as the right kidney and aorta. Gallstones may be found by ultrasonography in up to 30% of symptomatic patients with a negative oral cholecystogram.

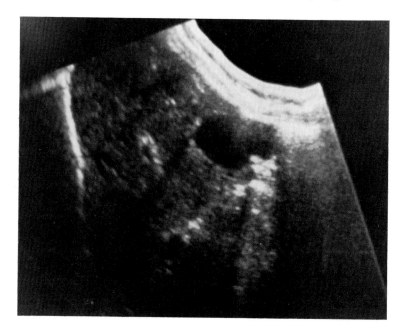

Fig. 3.3 Gallstones cause a clear acoustic shadow on ultrasound.

Upper gastrointestinal endoscopy

Endoscopy is widely used as the investigation of first choice in patients with suspected disease of the oesophagus, stomach and duodenum (Fig. 3.4). It can be carried out promptly with little discomfort in patients of all ages (Fig. 3.5). It is usually performed on an out-patient basis, using intravenous sedation, usually diazepam 5-20 mg. It is important to stress that patients who have been given intravenous diazepam should not drive a motor vehicle or operate dangerous machinery for 24 hours after the endoscopy; they must not drive themselves home from the examination.

Fibreoptic endoscopy is the diagnostic method of choice for the assessment of all mucosal lesions of oesophagus, stomach and duodenum: in particular it allows the taking of biopsies and cytology specimens from suspected malignant lesions. All gastric ulcers should be examined by endoscopy to exclude malignancy.

Upper gastrointestinal endoscopy constitutes a major and increasing part of the workload of the gastrointestinal investigation unit and because of this not all units are prepared to accept direct GP referrals. Many consultants will, however, accept a patient directly for endoscopy on the evidence provided in a well-written letter clearly indicating the patient's symptoms, in particular a patient with a radiological abnormality requiring further evaluation.

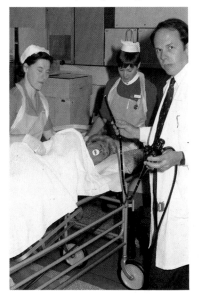 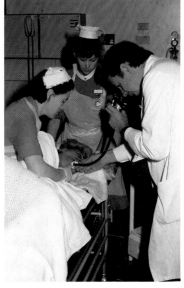

Fig. 3.4 A modern fibreoptic endoscope.

Fig. 3.5 Endoscopy is usually well tolerated.

Endoscopic examination of biliary and pancreatic ducts (endoscopic retrograde cholangiopancreatography) may be an appropriate investigation in patients complaining of 'indigestion', particularly if there is a history of biliary surgery or an elevated alkaline phosphatase.

MANAGEMENT

Duodenal ulcer

Specific dietary advice should be confined to eating regularly and avoiding specific foods that are known by the patient to aggravate symptoms. Other so-called 'ulcer' diets have not been shown to be helpful. Patients should be advised to stop smoking and to use paracetamol rather than aspirin as an analgesic.

The H_2-receptor antagonists, cimetidine and ranitidine, reduce gastric acidity and accelerate the healing of duodenal ulcers. Cimetidine 400 mg bd and ranitidine 150 mg bd have both been shown to be more effective than placebo. It is important that the last dose of each agent should be taken on retiring and not with the evening meal. While symptomatic relief may be obtained in the first week or two, it is probably important to continue therapy for four to six weeks (probably the latter) to ensure ulcer healing. Over 90% of duodenal ulcers will be healed by six weeks.

Lesser degrees of dyspeptic symptoms in patients with duodenal ulcer can be treated with antacids and these should be taken in an effective dose, e.g. 10-20 ml of a liquid preparation, one and three hours after food and at night. The taking of food initially buffers gastric acidity but this effect wears off after 60-90 minutes.

Treatment with H_2-receptor antagonists has not altered the natural history of duodenal ulceration. They are a treatment for duodenal ulceration, not a cure. Duodenal ulceration is a chronic disease: the majority of patients can be expected to relapse after treatment. However, as most will have only between one and three attacks a year it is preferable to treat each attack separately, as outlined above. In those patients who relapse more frequently, or relapse soon after stopping treatment, maintenance treatment should be considered. A single night-time dose of an H_2-receptor antagonist, either cimetidine 400 mg or ranitidine 150 mg, is highly effective (Fig. 3.6).

Most patients with duodenal ulcer can be expected to relapse

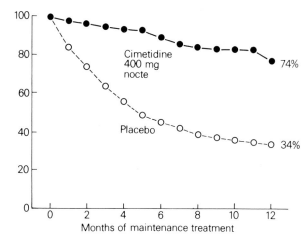

Fig. 3.6 Cimetidine 400 mg at bedtime prevents ulcer relapse in most patients.

Two other agents also speed the healing of duodenal ulceration: both are thought to work by coating the ulcer crater, protecting it from acid and pepsin attack. The first is tripotassium di-citrato bismuthate. It is taken as either a suspension (5 ml added to 15 ml of water) or a tablet, 30 minutes before meals and two hours after the last meal of the day. Milk and protein foods must be avoided for half an hour after ingestion. This compound should not be used for long-term maintenance treatment, owing to the fear that bismuth accumulation may cause central nervous system damage. The second compound is sucralfate, an aluminium-sucrose compound. A 1 g tablet is taken four times a day, again on an empty stomach so that the compound may coat any ulceration. Both these compounds appear to be effective for the management of acute peptic ulceration, but the depth of scientific understanding about their effectiveness and mechanism of action is much more limited than experience with the H_2-receptor antagonists.

Pirenzepine is a complex tricyclic compound derived from the benzodiazepine group. It is reported to exhibit a selective antimuscarinic effect, inhibiting gastric secretion without affecting visual accomodation, salivary flow or bladder function. Healing rates in clinical trials have been significantly greater than placebo, but less than those obtained with the H_2-receptor antagonists. The dose is 50 mg twice daily, and on this regimen some patients have reported anticholinergic side-effects.

Duodenal ulceration is a relapsing disease, running a chronic course, and it is important to make a definitive diagnosis by endoscopy or radiology before embarking on long-term treatment. It is particularly important to differentiate between duodenal ulcer and other conditions, including gastric carcinoma. Once a precise diagnosis of duodenal ulceration has been made, further investigation is not required unless the symptom pattern changes or the patient does not respond to treatment. The great majority of patients do not require repeated endoscopic examinations or barium meals. Most gastroenterologists recommend surgery only for the complications of duodenal ulcer - perforation, pyloric stenosis or haemorrhage (Fig. 3.7).

Gastric ulcer

The same general advice applies to gastric ulcer as to duodenal ulcer. It is important that patients with this condition do not smoke and that, if possible, they take no aspirin or non-

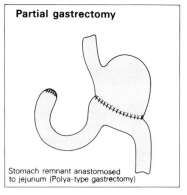

Partial gastrectomy

Stomach remnant anastomosed to jejunum (Polya-type gastrectomy)

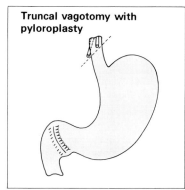

Truncal vagotomy with pyloroplasty

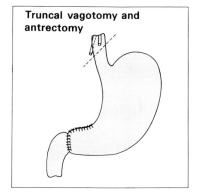

Truncal vagotomy and antrectomy

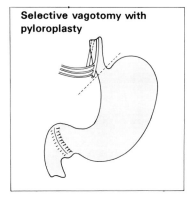

Selective vagotomy with pyloroplasty

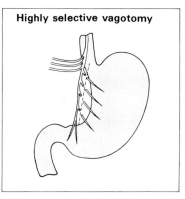

Highly selective vagotomy

Fig. 3.7 Surgical procedures for duodenal ulceration.

steroidal anti-inflammatory drugs. The same drugs that speed the healing of duodenal ulcers are also effective in the treatment of gastric ulcers. Gastric ulcers vary in surface area and depth and may be much larger than the more superficial duodenal ulcers. It is not surprising, therefore, that treatment may have to be continued for a much longer period to achieve complete healing. Whilst many small ulcers may heal within four weeks, larger ulcers may require 8-12 weeks of treatment.

Carbenoxolone sodium was commonly used for the treatment of gastric ulcer with good effect. Its steroidal side-effects (salt and water retention, with the production of hypokalaemia) make it inadvisable to use this agent in patients with heart disease or hypertension; indeed, the blood pressure and plasma potassium of patients treated with carbenoxolone should be monitored regularly.

It is important that gastric ulcers are biopsied to differentiate gastric carcinoma from benign ulceration. Any ulcer that is slow to heal or fails to heal should be re-biopsied. Gastric ulcers which fail to heal or which relapse after treatment are better treated surgically where the patient's general condition permits. Alternatively, maintenance treatment with cimetidine 400 mg nocte is effective.

Any gastric ulcer which fails to heal or heals only slowly should be re-biopsied

Gastric carcinoma

Gastric carcinoma has an appalling prognosis unless it is diagnosed at a very early stage. The five-year survival for all

Gastric carcinoma has an appalling prognosis unless diagnosed at an early stage

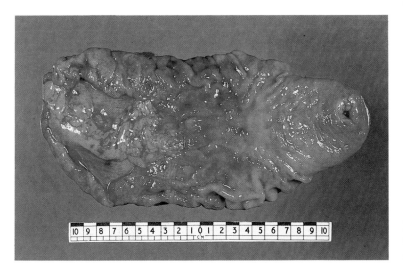

Fig. 3.8 Palliative surgical resection of advanced gastric cancer.

patients with gastric carcinoma is approximately 4%, whereas it is approximately 60% for patients who receive radical surgery of early gastric cancer. It is obvious that we should strive to achieve such early diagnosis, but the problem is that superficial gastric carcinoma can easily be confused with a minor benign gastric ulcer. The smaller the gastric ulcer, the more aggressive the investigation should be. Most patients with gastric malignancy require surgery, even if it is only palliative to relieve obstruction or to prevent chronic blood loss (Fig. 3.8).

Gallstones

Medical therapy of gallstones is suitable for only a minority of patients

The medical therapy of cholelithiasis, using chenodeoxycholate or ursodeoxycholate, is suitable for only a minority of patients. They must have radiolucent stones in a functioning gallbladder. Even if these stones do dissolve, they usually recur rapidly after cessation of treatment. Patients with symptomatic cholelithiasis usually require elective cholecystectomy.

FURTHER READING

Bouchier IAD (1983) Brides of quietness: silent gallstones. Br Med J 6: 415-416.

Feely J, Wormsley KG (1983) H_2-receptor antagonists: cimetidine and ranitidine. Br Med J 286: 695-697.

Geat MWL, Barnes RJ (1980) Endoscopic studies of dyspepsia in a general practice. Br Med J 2: 1136-1137.

Langman MJS (1982) What is happening to peptic ulcer? Br Med J 284: 1063-1064.

Leading Article (1982) Cimetidine and ranitidine. Lancet 2: 601-602.

Leading Article (1981) Gastric ulcer: benign or malignant? Br Med J 282: 843.

Littman A (1983) Cimetidine works for gastric ulcer, and more. N Engl J Med 308: 1356-1357.

Review Article (1982) Ranitidine and cimetidine in peptic ulcer. Drug Ther Bull 20: 57-59.

Thompson H (1982) Gastric cancer. Br Med J 284: 684-685.

Welch CE, Malt RA (1983) Abdominal surgery, part 1. N Engl J Med 308: 624-632.

E. SWARBRICK

Doctor, I often feel sick and vomit

4

Vomiting is the forceful ejection of gastric contents and is usually preceded or accompanied by nausea, the premonition of impending vomiting. Nausea commonly occurs without vomiting. Nausea and vomiting are frequently accompanied by hypersalivation, dysrrhythmias and defaecation. They may occur with diseases of all systems, but they are usually associated with other symptoms which help in making the correct diagnosis.

Vomiting is the forceful ejection of gastric contents

DIFFERENTIAL DIAGNOSIS

Nausea or vomiting may not be due to any form of gastrointestinal disease. Severe pain such as renal or biliary colic or fever from any cause, particularly in children, may provoke vomiting. Nausea and vomiting may be the only symptoms of a urinary tract infection or pneumonia, particularly in the elderly. Early-morning vomiting is universally recognised as one of the earliest signs of pregnancy. The oral contraceptive pill may induce a similar syndrome, although it is less common with the low-dose oestrogen pills.

Dysphagia is the usual presenting symptom of oesophageal strictures whether benign or malignant, although it is often associated with regurgitation of recently swallowed food (see Chapter 2). Similarly, the gastric contents refluxed by patients with hiatus hernia may simulate vomiting, but patients are usually aware of the difference between passive regurgitation and actual vomiting when questioned carefully (see Chapter 1).

Nausea and vomiting may be the only symptoms of a peptic ulcer, but it is usually associated with pain; vomiting frequently relieves this pain. Gastric carcinoma may present in a similar way. The cardinal symptom of pyloric obstruction is,

Table 4.1 Causes of chronic nausea and vomiting

Gastrointestinal
Peptic ulcer
Gastritis
Pyloric stenosis
Post-gastrectomy syndrome
Gastric carcinoma

Metabolic
Drugs
Pregnancy (or 'the pill')
Hypercalcaemia
Uraemia

Neuropsychiatric
Migraine
Vestibular disturbances
Psychogenic vomiting

of course, large-volume vomiting, but gastric stasis may also occur without obstruction in coeliac disease or diabetes.

Nausea and vomiting may also be caused by gastritis, whether the primary cause is alcohol, nicotine, drugs or unknown. Recurrent vomiting is a frequent complication of gastric surgery. Chronic pancreatitis usually presents as episodes of severe epigastric pain, radiating to the back, with vomiting.

If nausea and vomiting are associated with acute hepatitis and colitis, they usually reflect the severity of the primary illness. Furthermore, as in gastroenteritis, the symptoms are rarely chronic.

A number of metabolic disturbances are associated with vomiting. Nausea and vomiting may be an early presenting feature of uraemia, hypercalcaemia and the hyponatraemia found in Addison's disease. Many drugs cause nausea, notably digoxin, sulphonamides, sulphasalazine, tetracycline, metronidazole, aspirin, chemotherapeutic agents and narcotic analgesics.

Neurological causes of vomiting include migraine and disturbances of the balance. The vomiting associated with raised intracranial pressure is a late symptom; it is not usually associated with nausea.

Chronic or recurrent vomiting, without other symptoms, is commonly psychogenic and may be associated with anxiety. Such anxiety may be appropriate or inappropriate, depending upon the patient's personality and the stresses that are being imposed. It is frequently habit-forming and may be difficult to treat. There may be a history of similar symptoms in childhood or a family history of 'nervous stomach' or the irritable bowel syndrome. The vomiting associated with anorexia nervosa or anorexia bulimia is usually denied.

CLUES FROM THE HISTORY

Obtain information about the timing of nausea, associated pain, any systemic symptoms and the nature of the vomitus

A detailed history will be the best guide to diagnosis. It is most important to obtain information on the timing of nausea, associated pain, any systemic symptoms and the nature of the vomitus. The past medical history and a social history are often relevant.

Timing

Early-morning vomiting is a symptom associated with pregnancy. It usually starts after the first missed period and has disappeared by the beginning or the middle of the second trimester. Its cause is unknown and the most important response from the doctor is reassurance. Hyperemesis gravidarum is a rare but serious condition in which the vomiting is so severe that it causes dehydration and electrolyte disturbance. It may persist into the second half of pregnancy, but usually stops before then. There are no obvious reasons why the vomiting of pregnancy should become so serious in some women, except that there may be a strong psychological element, and there is often a previous history of emotional vomiting. The salt, water and potassium depletion may require replacement therapy. Antiemetics are often of little help.

Patients with alcoholic gastritis frequently vomit in the early morning and the vomitus is usually of small volume and mucoid; it may contain flecks of blood. 'Dry heaves', particularly induced by cleaning the teeth, usually indicate an alcohol problem. The nausea and vomiting associated with raised intracranial pressure and uraemia or occurring after a gastrectomy also tend to occur in the morning, rather than at other times.

'Dry heaves' usually indicate an alcohol problem

Nausea and vomiting are often related to meal times. There are two major patterns: early nausea and vomiting, which starts immediately before or even during a meal, and late vomiting, which comes hours after. The first is usually due to psychogenic causes; it is interesting that patients will sometimes rush dramatically from the table to vomit, but somehow always manage to reach the sink or lavatory. By contrast, vomiting due to organic disease may be uncontrollable. Care must be taken to differentiate regurgitation of food or drink during the meal, due to oesophageal disease, from vomiting. Nausea is not a feature of regurgitation and there is usually a clear history of dysphagia.

Late vomiting after a meal, occurring one to several hours later, suggests some form of gastric stasis, due either to organic obstruction, as in pyloric stenosis, or to functional stasis, as in post-vagotomy vomiting, diabetic neuropathy or coeliac disease. A milder disturbance of gastric emptying is described by patients who cannot finish a meal because they feel 'full up', or develop epigastric fullness and distension for some hours after a meal. Usually no organic cause is found for the symptoms, but they often respond to metoclopramide or domperidone.

Associated pain

'Indigestion' and dyspepsia should be carefully explored because it can mean very different things to different people. It is essential to differentiate heartburn from epigastric, central or lower abdominal pain. The pain of peptic ulcer is almost always felt in the epigastrium and possibly in the back; it is not felt periumbilically or diffusely in the abdomen. The single finger pointing to the epigastrium makes a peptic ulcer very likely, particularly if the symptoms occur at mealtimes, induce night waking and are relieved by antacids or cimetidine. Such pain is often relieved by vomiting. A past history of typical peptic ulcer pain, with appropriate symptoms, may point to a diagnosis of pyloric stenosis.

Epigastric pain associated with severe back pain and vomiting may suggest a posterior duodenal ulcer or pancreatic disease, particularly chronic pancreatitis or a carcinoma.

The severe, epigastric, constant pain of biliary colic, which induces sweating and an inability to keep still, often improves shortly after the patient has vomited. Central colicky abdominal pain, associated with gurgling and copious vomiting of bile-stained fluid, suggests intestinal obstruction. Patients rarely vomit with large bowel obstruction until late in the illness, when marked distension and absolute constipation should facilitate the diagnosis.

Systemic symptoms

Anorexia is rarely a helpful symptom, as it almost invariably accompanies nausea. Indeed a normal appetite associated with vomiting should raise suspicion of a psychogenic cause. Unless associated with hyperthyroidism or widely disseminated malignant disease, weight loss is due to anorexia and a reduced food intake. Constipation frequently accompanies nausea and vomiting, owing to reduced food intake and dehydration. Weight gain may suggest that there is no serious organic cause for the nausea and vomiting but some patients with peptic ulcer disease put on weight because of continually nibbling to relieve symptoms.

Normal appetite associated with vomiting suggests a psychogenic cause

The vomitus

The contents of the vomitus may give some clue to its aetiology. The diagnosis of gastric stasis is suggested if the vomitus contains food taken hours or even days previously.

Patients may recognise certain vegetables or salad items, such as sweetcorn or tomato skins. The presence of bile in the vomit is of little help, unless large volumes of bile-stained fluid are being vomited, which should warn of impending dehydration. Vomit which smells faecal suggests a small bowel obstruction or an ileus, a gastrocolic fistula or gastric stasis with secondary bacterial overgrowth. All require urgent investigation.

The vomiting of blood is potentially serious (see Chapter 5). If blood first appears after several vomits, the bleeding may be due to mucosal damage at or about the oesophagogastric junction. This will include the long linear tears of the Mallory-Weiss syndrome (Fig. 4.1), but also minor mucosal damage to the gastric fundus.

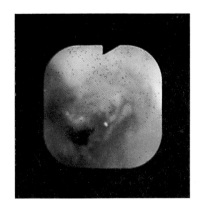

Fig. 4.1   A Mallory Weiss mucosal tear in the upper stomach seen at endoscopy.

Past medical history

Details of previous surgery are obviously important. Information on childhood health may be very illuminating if psychogenic causes are suspected. While 'little bellyachers' may not always become 'big bellyachers', patients with psychogenic vomiting will frequently have been 'sickly children'. There is frequently a family history of 'nervous tummy' or of being 'gastric'. However, peptic ulcers, gallstones, coeliac disease and inflammatory bowel disease tend to be familial.

Social history

Information about home, job, marriage, children and sexual problems may be particularly relevant. Knowledge of these areas, with some assessment of the degree of anxiety that each or any of these may produce, will indicate the appropriateness of emotional responses in a patient. Some anxiety is often justifiable; being 'sick with fear' has an excellent prognosis, provided the stress factors can be removed or go away. However, anxiety in others may be inappropriate and chronic; the symptoms will be harder to treat and the prognosis less good.

ABNORMALITIES ON EXAMINATION

The physical examination is often disappointingly unhelpful and the main clues to the diagnosis will be in the history. Nevertheless, a thorough open-minded examination is essential if a diagnosis of organic disease is not be missed or delayed.

Weight loss and cachexia, jaundice or lymphadenopathy will have obvious implications.

Abdominal examination may reveal distension, scars, visible peristalsis, tenderness or a mass. Examination of hernial orifices may reveal the cause of intestinal obstruction (Fig. 4.2). The classic sign of pyloric stenosis is a succussion splash, and it is sometimes possible to see gastric peristalsis. Distorsion and tinkling bowel sounds indicate intestinal obstruction.

Painless vomiting may be due to raised intracranial pressure; it is sensible to check for papilloedema, nystagmus and cranial nerve abnormalities.

INVESTIGATIONS

The investigations employed in the patient with nausea and vomiting are esssentially simple, and depend upon the likely diagnosis based on history and examination.

All patients should have a full blood count, urea, electrolytes and liver function tests. A full blood count may reveal anaemia (see Chapter 16); iron deficiency would probably be due to some form of peptic or malignant ulceration, or to disease of the small bowel. A raised MCV may be due to folate or vitamin B12 deficiency, or to liver disease, most commonly alcoholic in origin. Urea and electrolyte disturbances may arise secondary to continuing vomiting; they may be severe,

Fig. 4.2 Two patients with incarcerated inguinal herniae causing intestinal obstruction.

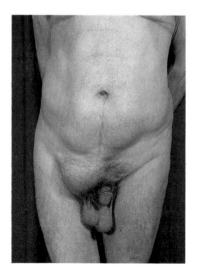
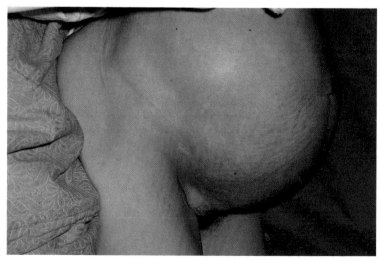

particularly in gastric stasis, intestinal obstruction or hyperemesis gravidarum. Nausea and vomiting may be the presenting symptom of uraemia. A plasma calcium estimation should be performed routinely as hypercalcaemia may first present as painless vomiting. Elevation of liver transaminases and gamma glutamyl transpeptidase may also help in the diagnosis of an occult alcohol problem. If there is marked back pain with the vomiting, the serum amylase should be estimated to identify acute or relapsing pancreatitis.

A barium swallow and meal are frequently indicated for the investigation of nausea and vomiting: good quality double-contrast films are essential. If there is gastric stasis of barium, the degree of duodenal filling is a useful way to differentiate pyloric stenosis (Fig. 4.3) from gastric atony or high small bowel obstructions.

If no diagnosis has been made after these primary investigations, and an organic cause is suspected, the patient should probably be referred for a specialist opinion,

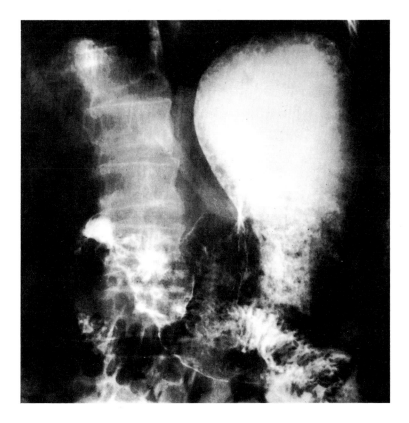

Fig. 4.3 Pyloric stenosis causing retention of old food mixed with barium.

particularly for upper intestinal endoscopy. In some centres gastroduodenoscopy has replaced the barium meal, but this will depend upon the interest and expertise of the hospital team. Some feel that endoscopy can use up so much clinical time that the diagnostic benefits over a barium study do not justify its routine use; they reserve endoscopy for special problems. Others feel that it is better to use the most accurate investigation as the primary procedure. The barium meal is actually better in the diagnosis of gastric stasis and upper gastrointestinal obstruction (Fig. 4.4): it shows overall anatomy and there is no hazard from aspiration of vomitus. Alternatively, only endoscopy can identify bile reflux through the pylorus and into the stomach, with resultant fiery gastritis. Endoscopy is more likely to produce the correct diagnosis.

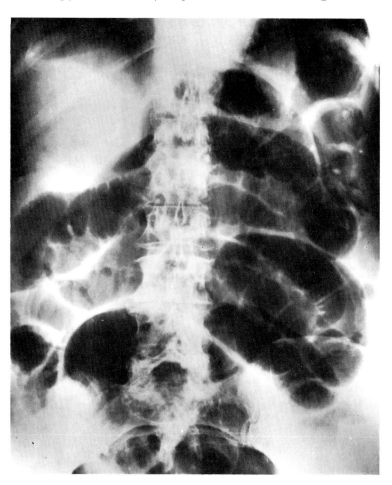

Fig. 4.4 Intestinal obstruction with dilated loops of small bowel shown on a plain abdominal X-ray.

MANAGEMENT

The surgical treatment of pyloric stenosis should not be delayed; it usually alleviates the secondary nausea and vomiting.

The cure for gastritis induced by nicotine, drugs or alcohol is self-apparent, but such abstention is often difficult, and some symptomatic measures may be needed, either an antacid or an antiemetic, or both.

Nausea and vomiting due to certain drugs, such as sulphasalazine or digoxin, may merely reflect overdosage and reduction of the dose may relieve symptoms. Drug-induced vomiting can be extremely difficult to treat if use of the drug is essential, for example an antimetabolite for malignant disease or a narcotic analgesic for severe pain.

Many doctors prescribe parenteral phenothiazine antiemetics simultaneously with a narcotic analgesic (perphenazine 5 mg or prochlorperazine 12.5 mg). Major sedation with massive doses of antiemetics may be needed to control vomiting caused by anti-cancer drugs. This prophylactic use of antiemetics is generally more effective than trying to control nausea or vomiting after they have started.

Massive doses of antiemetics may be necessary to control the vomiting caused by anti-cancer drugs

The type of drug used for the relief of acute nausea and vomiting depends, to some extent, upon the aetiology of the upset. Antihistamines are extremely useful for the treatment of vestibular disturbances and travel sickness; in terms of their antiemetic properties there is little to choose between the preparations (cinnarizine, cyclizine, dimenhydrinate or promethazine). However, such drugs have sedative side effects, causing a variable degree of somnolence in different individuals. Patients should be warned of this fact; it may be useful to experiment to see which drug is best suited to an individual patient. Cinnarizine has been found to be very useful for sea sickness and seems to cause less sedation than others. The recommended dose is 15-30 mg, up to three times daily. The first dose should be taken prophylactically if possible. Phenothiazines and metoclopramide are ineffective for motion sickness.

Cinnarizine is useful for sea sickness

In nausea and vomiting due to causes other than disturbances of the labyrinthine apparatus phenothiazines are often the drug of choice. Prochlorperazine, perphenazine or trifluoperazine are all effective and possibly less sedating than chlorpromazine. The phenothiazine drugs may produce extrapyramidal side-effects, but these are not common when used in small doses for nausea and vomiting.

Metoclopramide is an effective and commonly used antiemetic, which is very useful for gastrointestinal causes of nausea and vomiting. It not only works as a central antiemetic, but its peripheral action causes speeding of gastric emptying. It is used in doses of 10 mg up to three times daily and can also be administered parenterally. Approximately 1% of patients will develop extrapyramidal symptoms and signs: an acute and most frightening oculogyric crisis can be controlled by an injection of atropine. Some patients taking metoclopramide will notice an unpleasant restlessness of the legs. Domperidone has effects similar to those of metoclopramide, but does not have central nervous system side-effects.

Nausea and vomiting in the first trimester of pregnancy seldom require any drug therapy

The nausea and vomiting in the first trimester of pregnancy do not usually require drug therapy. All drug therapy should be avoided if possible, but if the vomiting becomes severe, it may be necessary to resort to the use of an antihistamine or phenothiazine.

FURTHER READING

Albibi R, McCallum W (1983) Metoclopramide: pharmacology and clinical application. Ann Intern Med 98: 86-95.

Review Article (1983) Domperidone: a new anti-emetic. Drug Ther Bull 21: 47-48.

Review Article (1983) Drugs for travel sickness. Drug Ther Bull 19: 19-20.

Doctor, I've vomited blood!

5

Upper gastrointestinal haemorrhage is a common emergency accounting for 20,000 hospital admissions per year in England and Wales. In two-thirds there will have been a haematemesis. This means that a district general hospital serving a population of 300,000 will admit between two and four such patients a week.

The following important points may save time and unnecessary or incorrect referral and investigations.

1. *Was it really blood?* It is essential to confirm the patient's statement. Although usually obvious, patients and witnesses often get it wrong. Where possible inspect the vomit; is it red food matter rather than blood? The term 'coffee-ground' vomit is frequently used in error. If in doubt, test for occult blood. A rectal examination may demonstrate melaena.

Two important points: was it really blood and where did the blood come from

2. *Where did the blood come from?* Did the patient really vomit the blood or was it coughed up? Did it come from the mouth itself? Did the patient have a nose bleed?

DIFFERENTIAL DIAGNOSIS

In the course of the clinical assessment the following differential diagnoses must be borne in mind (Table 5.1).

Table 5.1 Causes of upper gastrointestinal haemorrhage

Common	*Less common*	*Rare*
Duodenal and gastric ulcer (together account for about 50% of all bleeds)	Varices	Benign gastric tumours
	Gastric carcinoma	Duodenal tumours
	Stomal ulcer	Arterial aneurysms
Acute gastric/duodenal erosions	Oesophageal ulcer	Pseudoxanthoma elasticum
Mallory Weiss tears	Oesophageal carcinoma	Hereditary haemorrhagic telangiectasia
Oesophagitis		Haemangiomas
		Bleeding disorders
		Spurious bleeding

Haematemesis most commonly results from duodenal or gastric ulceration.

GASTRIC OR DUODENAL ULCERATION. Haematemesis in the United Kingdom most commonly results from gastric or duodenal ulceration. Acute ulceration may frequently occur for no clear reason. Aspirin, non-steroidal anti-inflammatory agents and alcohol may cause acute ulceration in otherwise healthy patients. Acute ulceration is also seen in extremely ill patients, especially those with burns, renal failure or cirrhosis. Chronic peptic ulceration (Figs 5.1 to 5.4) is extremely common; 10% of the adult population have an ulcer before the age of 60. However, not uncommonly the vomiting of blood is the first symptom of ulceration, especially with gastric ulcers in the elderly.

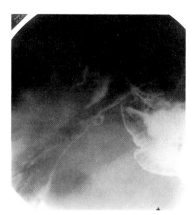

Fig. 5.1 An X-ray showing a benign gastric ulcer.

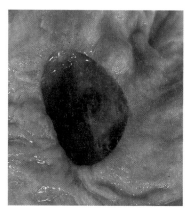

Fig. 5.2 An endoscopy view of a bleeding gastric ulcer.

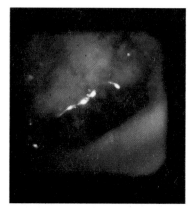

Fig. 5.3 An endoscopy view of a gastric ulcer with the stigmata of bleeding.

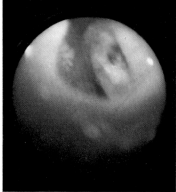

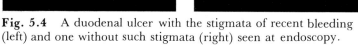

Fig. 5.4 A duodenal ulcer with the stigmata of recent bleeding (left) and one without such stigmata (right) seen at endoscopy.

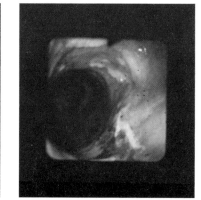

Fig. 5.5 Bleeding oesophagitis shown on endoscopy.

HIATUS HERNIA AND OESOPHAGITIS (Fig. 5.5). Hiatus hernias are common and there is a temptation to attribute bleeding to the hernia. Bleeding is in fact uncommon unless the hernia is associated with reflux oesophagitis (see Chapter 1). Rarely massive bleeding results from ulceration in a rolling type of hernia. Symptoms of heartburn and reflux accompany the former but not the latter. A chronic benign ulcer is occasionally found in the lower oesophagus, almost always in association with a columnar lining to the oesophagus (Barrett's ulcer) (Fig. 5.6).

MALLORY WEISS TEARS. These occur at the oesophagogastric junction and are probably much commoner than previously described. Violent vomiting or belching can cause this type of mucosal laceration.

It is uncommon for a hiatus hernia to cause haematemesis

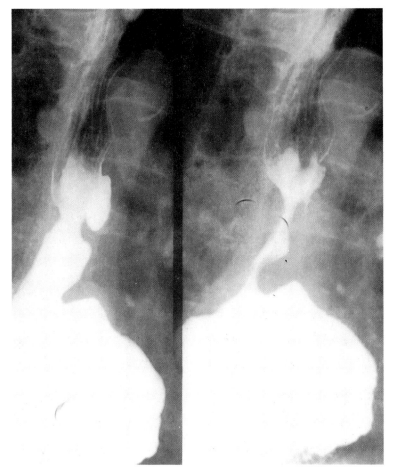

Fig. 5.6 An X-ray showing an oesophageal ulcer in a columnar-lined oesophagus.

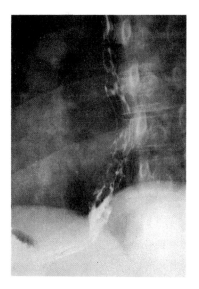

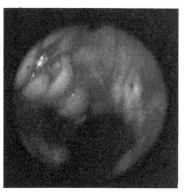

Fig. 5.7 Oesophageal varices shown on X-ray and on endoscopy.

OESOPHAGEAL VARICES (Fig. 5.7). Bleeding from oesophageal varices is common in the United States and France, but much less common in the United Kingdom. However, as alcohol consumption increases in this country this situation is changing.

CARCINOMA OF STOMACH. Acute bleeding occurs in only 10% of patients with gastric carcinoma.

ARTERIAL ANEURYSM. Aneurysms of the abdominal aorta, usually adjacent to the third part of the duodenum, may rupture into the gastrointestinal tract, causing a spectacular haemorrhage.

SPURIOUS BLEEDING. It is wise to be alert to this rare but well recognised cause of 'bleeding'. Self-inflicted trauma may be a cause of bleeding and is a form of the Munchausen syndrome.

CLUES FROM THE HISTORY

About 30% of patients with peptic ulcers are asymptomatic before the bleed and 50% of all patients who bleed have no symptoms relevant to the cause of the bleeding. Although sometimes unhelpful, a careful history may provide useful clues to the cause of the bleeding; the following points should be covered.

DRUGS. Few patients are taking no drugs at all, and many are taking medications that have been associated with gastrointestinal bleeding. In very few instances, however, is the association beyond doubt. Non-steroidal anti-inflammatory drugs are the most notorious; they are undoubtedly a potent cause of indigestion, ulceration and serious bleeding. There is no definite evidence that oral steroids cause ulceration. Anticoagulants will cause bleeding, but probably only in the presence of a pre-existing gastrointestinal lesion.

OCCUPATION. Occupations disposed to a high alcohol intake, such as barmen, hoteliers or publicans, should alert one to the possibility of bleeding varices. A high level of suspicion for this diagnosis is important, as the management is quite different from that of other causes of upper gastrointestinal bleeding.

PAST HISTORY. Enquire about peptic ulceration and indigestion, past and present; previous abdominal surgery; previous haematemesis and melaena; and pointers to a bleeding diathesis, such as nose bleeds, bruising or a bleeding tendency such as haemophilia.

ALCOHOL CONSUMPTION. Answers are frequently misleading.

VOMITING. In most haematemeses blood is present from the outset. The exception is the Mallory Weiss syndrome, where blood appears at the end of a vomiting spell; as it comes from the lower oesophagus, the blood is characteristically bright.

MALIGNANCY. Weight loss, dysphagia and anorexia raise the possibility of carcinoma.

ABNORMALITIES ON EXAMINATION

There are two objectives of the examination: first, to assess the haemodynamic state of the patient to determine the degree of shock, and, second, to make a diagnosis. The first is by far the most important in the short term. Clinical examination is usually unhelpful in establishing the diagnosis.

First resuscitate, then make a diagnosis

Assessment of the haemodynamic status

Tachycardia and hypotension indicate hypovolaemia, which signifies acute blood loss. In general, a systolic blood pressure of less than 100 mmHg and a pulse greater than 100/minute indicate a 20% depletion of blood volume. With more serious blood loss the signs of shock -- peripheral constriction, fast thready pulse, sweating, pallor and profound hypotension --demand urgent on-the-spot resuscitation and immediate transfer to hospital.

Diagnostic clues

Fig. 5.8 Stomal ulceration.

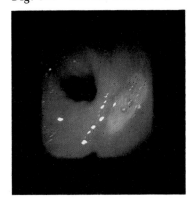

The presence of anaemia indicates chronic blood loss: in the early stage of haemorrhage the patient is not anaemic as haemodilution has not occurred.

Signs of chronic liver disease, such as liver palms, spider naevi, jaundice, hepatosplenomegaly or ascites, suggest liver disease. Oesophageal varices are likely if the spleen can be palpated (see Chapter 11).

Emaciation, lymphadenopathy, a hard irregular liver or abdominal masses may point to underlying malignancy.

Bruising and purpura suggest a bleeding disorder.

Abdominal scars may have been omitted from the history. They need to be identified as they may be highly relevant to the cause of the bleeding and to any possible surgery which may ensue (Fig. 5.8).

INITIAL ACTION BY THE GP

Any patient who has bled acutely within the last 48 hours should be admitted to hospital for observation. It is not possible to identify those patients who may bleed again. Patients who have bled a substantial amount, and in particular those showing signs of hypovolaemia and shock, need urgent referral to the nearest casualty department. Where circumstances permit, an intravenous line should be established, if only to provide 0.9% saline. If plasma expanders are available these can be commenced after blood has been taken for grouping and cross-matching. The patient may need to be accompanied to hospital by the doctor to supervise resuscitation during transit. If not actively bleeding, the patient should be transferred wherever possible to a gastrointestinal unit equipped for endoscopy.

Particular care is needed with elderly patients. The mortality from upper gastrointestinal bleeding is less than 1% in those under 40 and greater than 20% in those over 80 years of age. The elderly compensate much less well for acute falls in blood volume. They are much more prone to cardiac and renal complications than younger patients. They are also more vulnerable to over-transfusion and have a higher mortality rate from any subsequent surgery.

Only rarely will a bleeding patient be investigated on an out-patient basis. Full blood count, platelet count, prothrombin time and blood grouping are required; serum should be saved in case transfusion is required. However, such a patient will almost certainly need hospital investigation to determine the site of the haemorrhage.

A proposed management plan for the patient with haematemesis is given in Fig. 5.9.

INVESTIGATIONS

On arrival at hospital the first priority is to resuscitate the patient but the following investigations (Table 5.2) are required:

1. Full blood count including platelets.
2. Prothrombin time.
3. Blood group and cross-match: sufficient should be cross-matched for the treatment of shock, correction of anaemia and a reserve to be held for 48 hours in case of a further bleed.

Any patient who has bled acutely within the last 48 hours should be admitted to hospital

---

Particular care is needed with elderly patients

Table 5.2   Investigations in a patient with gastrointestinal bleeding

Urgent
Haematological:
  haemoglobin
  platelets
  blood group (and save serum)
  cross match
  prothrombin time
Diagnostic:
  endoscopy
  barium meal (if
    endoscopy not available)

Additional (especially if
  surgery is contemplated)
Urea and electrolytes
Liver function tests
HBsAG (if liver disease is
  suspected)
Chest X-ray
ECG

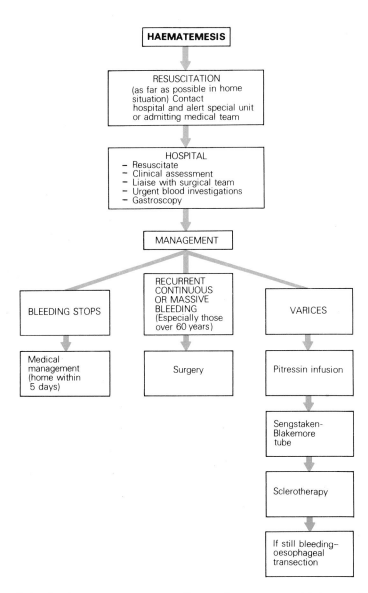

Fig. 5.9 A management plan for a patient with haematemesis.

It is also important to assess fitness for surgery which may be necessary at any time in the next few days; this is particularly so with elderly patients who should have a chest X-ray and ECG on admission. Occult liver disease must be excluded by liver function tests. However, if liver disease is suspected, the hepatitis B antigen (HBsAg, Australia antigen) must be tested on admission to protect hospital staff exposed to the patient's blood.

Endoscopy or barium meal?

The choice of first-line diagnostic procedure rests between endoscopy and double-contrast barium meal, both of which are available in most teaching or district general hospitals. Although endoscopy is now generally accepted to be diagnostically superior, it has not rendered the barium meal redundant. Both investigations may be necessary, especially where the diagnosis is uncertain.

The great advantage of endoscopy is direct visualisation in colour, enabling confident identification of the bleeding site. Although frequently not bleeding at the time of endoscopy, the source of the haemorrhage can often be identified by the black base of an ulcer or an adherent clot over a protruding artery (Figs 5.1 to 5.5). These signs of recent bleeding often identify the patient at particular risk of re-bleeding.

Superficial lesions, erosions, oesophagitis or Mallory Weiss tears can be identified with far greater accuracy during endoscopy. In addition there is the facility for biopsy where malignancy is suspected (Figs 5.10, 5.11) and direct application of haemostatic techniques where appropriate.

Signs of recent bleeding identify the patient at risk of re-bleeding

---

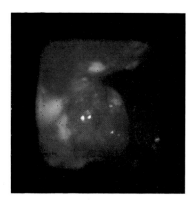

Fig. 5.10   Gastric carcinoma shown on X-ray and on endoscopy.

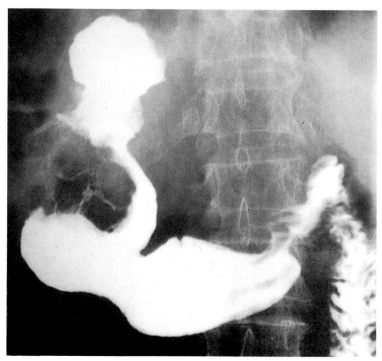

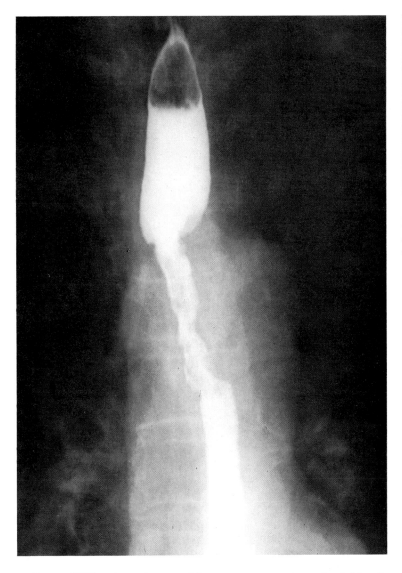

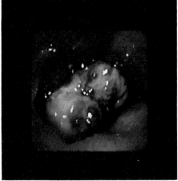

Fig. 5.11 Oesophageal carcinoma shown on X-ray and on endoscopy.

Some 30% of patients with upper gastrointestinal bleeds have two lesions on barium meal, but endoscopy can often identify which one has been bleeding. Of patients with oesophageal varices who bleed, 60% bleed from a site other than the varices; this can only be established endoscopically.

However, it should be remembered that endoscopy may cause recurrence of bleeding or allow inhalation of gastric contents, especially in the restless patient with a stomach full of blood. Furthermore, where bleeding is continuing and excessive, the procedure may be positively harmful, providing no information and delaying inevitable surgical intervention.

Unless endoscopy is performed early after the bleed, much of its advantage is lost because superficial erosions and tears may heal within 24-48 hours. The diagnostic rate falls from 80-90% if endoscopy is carried out within 12 hours of a bleed to 50% if endoscopy is carried out two days after the event.

The difficult bleeder

Some patients who bleed defy diagnosis. Where endoscopy has been unhelpful radiology is required to look not only at the upper gastrointestinal tract but also at the small bowel. This may also be unhelpful. A thorough search of the nasopharynx by an ENT specialist may be indicated. Mesenteric angiography may demonstrate abnormal collections of vessels indicating a tumour or vascular malformation. Occasionally laparotomy is carried out as an absolute last resort. The use of a flexible endoscope to examine the small bowel during surgery is a helpful adjunct to laparoscopy.

EMERGENCY MANAGEMENT

Very occasionally upper gastrointestinal haemorrhage will be investigated and treated on an out-patient basis or entirely by the general practitioner. Apart from the early resuscitation, the principles of treatment are the same, whether treatment is initiated in hospital or out of hospital.

Resuscitation

The aim of the exercise is to keep the patient alive! It is no good having a comprehensive history and accurate diagnosis, but a dead patient! The mortality rate from upper gastrointestinal haemorrhage is approximately 10%. Early effective resuscitation may be life-saving. The shocked or severely hypovolaemic patient needs volume replacement with whole blood as soon as available and a plasma expander in the meantime. Rapid correction of hypovolaemia is important and can be carried out more safely if monitored with a central venous pressure line. Where haemodynamic disturbance is not apparent a central line is not necessary, but a more cautious approach is required in the elderly and those with cardiac

Early effective resuscitation may be life-saving

disease. Circulatory overload can easily occur without close monitoring and heart failure may need treatment before the patient is transfused.

Transfusion

Patients need transfusion for two reasons: shock or anaemia. Any patient with a haemoglobin less than 10 g/dl should receive transfusion in case of further haemorrhage. As re-bleeding usually occurs within 48 hours of the first episode, a reserve of two units of blood should be kept available to cover that danger period. If more than 6 pints of blood are given the patient may require fresh frozen plasma and platelets to maintain haemostasis.

Reassurance

Vomiting blood is an extremely frightening experience. It is of great importance to reassure the patient and to keep the patient informed about what is happening. However, sedatives or morphine must not be given.

Sedatives or morphine must not be given after haematemesis

Non-surgical haemostatic techniques

Endoscopists are keen to find ways to treat a bleeding point, thereby controlling haemorrhage without involving the surgeon! Diathermy electrocoagulation or lasers may provide an answer in the future, but at present they are experimental.

Drugs

Although it is logical to give peptic ulcer healing drugs to patients with upper gastrointestinal haemorrhage to speed ulcer healing, there is no good evidence they prevent early re-bleeding or stop acute bleeding when given either orally or parenterally.

Surgery

The surgical team on call should be informed about all patients with serious upper gastrointestinal bleeds admitted under a physician, since the decision to operate may have to be made rapidly. Although surgery will be unnecessary for most patients, all should be considered as potential candidates for operation and assessed accordingly.

Indications for surgery are continued or recurrent bleeding. The patient's age is highly relevant in making the decision. The mortality rate from gastrointestinal bleeding is almost entirely confined to the elderly and the mortality rate increases fourfold when recurrent haemorrhage occurs after admission.

It is generally thought that surgery is more likely to have a successful outcome if carried out early before the patient's general condition deteriorates. However, most deaths from gastrointestinal haemorrhage occur during recovery from surgery. It is possible that early surgery may substitute death from haemorrhage with death from the stress of surgery.

> Early surgery may replace death from haemorrhage with death from the stress of surgery

Long-term treatment

Most patients who survive a substantial upper gastrointestinal haemorrhage will have some form of peptic ulcer, which will require effective medical treatment (see Chapter 3). All will require oral iron therapy to replenish their iron stores (see Chapter 16). Patients must be warned that the iron will discolour their stools, otherwise they may be alarmed that the melaena has recurred. All non-steroidal anti-inflammatory drugs should be stopped, if possible, and the patient should be warned against taking any remedies containing aspirin. No special diet is required. Alcohol in moderation is quite acceptable.

Oesophageal varices

Because the manangement of bleeding from varices is quite different from other forms of upper gastrointestinal bleeding, a high level of suspicion for its existence and accurate diagnosis is of the greatest importance. At least 60% of patients with varices who bleed, bleed from a site other than the varices (Fig. 5.12); inappropriate treatment by surgery should be avoided.

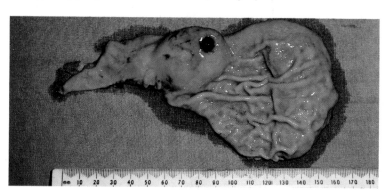

Fig. 5.12 Surgical diagnosis: bleeding leiomyoma of the stomach.

The initial mortality rate is high and depends principally on the state of the liver. Jaundice, ascites, a low albumin and a prolonged prothrombin time make the prognosis extremely poor.

If the hepatitis B surface antigen is positive (suspect homosexuals, drug addicts, haemophiliacs and those from the non-temperate areas of the world) the staff must take extra care, wearing gloves, gown and mask during nursing, diagnostic and therapeutic procedures.

HBsAG -- suspect homosexuals, drug addicts, haemophiliacs and foreigners

The patient with bleeding oesophageal varices needs standard resuscitation, but if bleeding continues pitressin is an effective means of arresting haemorrhage. All patients require standard prophylactic treatment for hepatic failure.

If pitressin fails, a Sengstaken-Blakemore tube (Fig. 5.13) can be used. Though unpleasant for the patient this tube, which incorporates compressive oesophageal and gastric balloons, is very effective in stopping bleeding, albeit often only temporarily.

Sclerotherapy is probably the most exciting and hopeful advance in the management of varices, with direct elimination of the varices via an endoscope. Surgical transection of the oesophagus, using a stapling gun, may also provide life-saving control of variceal haemorrhage.

Prognosis for the bleeding patient

It is disheartening that, despite major advances in diagnostic and therapeutic techniques, the mortality rate from

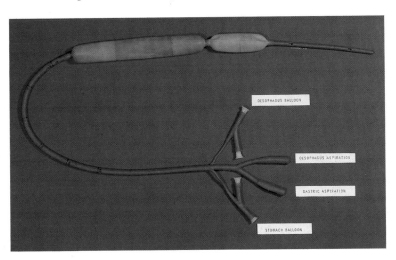

Fig. 5.13 A Sengstaken-Blakemore tube.

gastrointestinal haemorrhage has remained unchanged over the last twenty years. This fact demands a critical reassessment of medical and surgical management in these patients. The following factors have been shown to influence the prognosis.

Sixty seems the critical age above which mortality rises steeply. Under 40 years the mortality rate is less than 1%; from 60 to 79 years the mortality rate rises to 10% and above 80 years to over 20%.

Any serious medical disease, in particular, cardiovascular, pulmonary or renal disease, leads to a worse prognosis.

Bleeding from varices in general carries a very poor prognosis.

The prognosis is worse where large bleeds are accompanied by marked haemodynamic change and when recurrent bleeds occur.

Haematemesis as the presenting feature is associated with a higher mortality than melaena alone. Where bleeding occurs with a short history of symptoms, or with no preceding symptoms, the prognosis is worse.

It is clear that the young tend to survive and it is the elderly who die. This latter group is the one requiring the most meticulous care. The failure of the overall mortality rate to fall may reflect an increasingly ageing population.

Various studies have suggested that a conservative non-surgical approach to treatment should be pursued in those under 60, whilst a more aggressive approach to diagnosis and early surgery should be the policy in the elderly. It may be that doctors are disinclined to take such an approach in elderly, often frail, patients and this cautious approach may deny them the type of care which reduces mortality. On the other hand, those factors which increase mortality from bleeding also increase mortality from surgery, possibly off-setting the advantages of early surgery.

The expected benefits from earlier and more accurate diagnosis have not been realised and there is no doubt that in some circumstances the insistance on a diagnosis may delay effective medical and surgical treatment.

The best results, as measured by mortality rates, have been achieved in those hospitals with units which specialise in the care of the bleeding patient. Where there is a clear management policy and an experienced team, there exists the best hope for future improvement in survival from haematemesis and melaena.

FURTHER READING

Barker D, Ogilvie A, Henry D (1983) Cimetidine and tranexamic acid in the treatment of acute upper gastrointestinal tract bleeding. N Engl J Med 308: 1517-1575.

Cochrane P, McArthur P (1980) Medical and surgical management of upper gastrointestinal haemorrhage. Update 21: 1475-1487.

Chalmers DM (1977) Practical management of acute upper gastrointestinal haemorrhage. Hospital Update 313-323.

Dronfield MW, Langman MJS (1978) Acute upper gastrointestinal bleeding. Br J Hosp Med 197-108.

Korman MG (1982) Upper gastrointestinal haemorrhage. Medicine 1: 597-599.

Mayberry JF, Penny WJ, Counsell BR, Rhodes J (1981) Mortality in acute gastrointestinal haemorrhage: A six year survey from the University Hospital of Wales. Postgrad Med 57: 627-632.

Young AE (1982) Stopping the haemorrhage from peptic ulcers. Br Med J 284: 530.

Doctor, I've always got stomach ache

Patients complaining of abdominal pain over a period of years are common in general practice and in gastroenterology clinics. They are often a source of worry, frustration and confusion. Most chronic abdominal pain, however, is not due to organic disease. A major danger to such patients is the misapplication of organic remedies, principally surgery, to their functional problems.

DIFFERENTIAL DIAGNOSIS

Many of the well known causes of acute abdominal pain may also give rise to symptoms over a period of months or even years.

Peptic ulceration, reflux oesophagitis, biliary colic, recurrent acute or chronic pancreatitis, renal and ureteric colic, expanding or dissecting aortic aneurysms, Crohn's disease, pelvic inflammatory disease, low-grade intestinal obstruction, constipation, diverticular disease of the colon, endometriosis, myocardial ischaemia, and even rare disorders such as familial periodic Mediterranean fever, intestinal angina and paroxysmal nocturnal haemoglobinuria, all fall within the differential diagnosis.

However, by far the commonest cause of chronic abdominal pain is due to a functional, rather than organic, illness.

CLUES FROM THE HISTORY

The essence of dealing with patients with chronic abdominal pain is a precise history. This is often difficult to obtain because the patients have frequently seen many other doctors, and their

Table 6.1 Differential diagnosis of chronic or recurrent abdominal pain

Functional causes

Common organic causes
Peptic ulcer
Reflux oesophagitis
Gallstones
Pancreatitis
Crohn's disease
Pelvic inflammatory disease
Diverticular disease
Constipation
Renal colic

Uncommon organic causes
Aortic aneurysms
Intestinal obstruction
Endometriosis
Myocardial ischaemia
Familial Mediterranean fever
Intestinal angina
Paroxysmal nocturnal
   haemoglobinuria
Porphyria
Lead poisoning

Table 6.2 Abdominal pain history

Site
Radiation and referral
Timing
Duration
Modifying features
Associated features
Psychological background

The site of pain should be confirmed by examination

history has been embellished through repetition. Furthermore many patients find pain difficult to describe and need considerable help. The essential features are the site, radiation and referral of the pain, its nature, timing and duration, factors which modify the pain, and any associated features.

Site, radiation and referral of pain

The site, radiation and referral of pain should be confirmed on examination because seated patients often indicate a site of pain considerably remote from the actual area in which the pain is felt. Bizarre extra-abdominal pain referral is well recognised in both organic and functional abdominal problems. For instance, radiation to the thigh occurs with diseases of the testicle or ureter, but it also occurs in the irritable bowel syndrome. Radiation to the shoulder is characteristic of diaphragmatic irritation, but pain from the splenic flexure may also radiate from the left upper quadrant to the shoulder. The pain of biliary colic or pancreatic disease may be referred to the back, but this again applies equally to pain from the irritable bowel.

Nature of pain

The nature of the pain is important, although patients frequently find their pain difficult to describe. Impatience on the part of the doctor rarely helps. Certain diseases produce pain with distinct qualities. Well known examples are the burning or gnawing pain of duodenal ulcer, the cramping pain of intestinal obstruction, or the episodes of continuous severe epigastric pain associated with biliary colic. Biliary colic usually lasts a short time, but is so severe that the patient considers calling out the general practitioner or ringing for an ambulance. Although the intensity of abdominal pain is often roughly correlated with the seriousness of the underlying pathology, many patients with functional abdominal pain claim to have had years of indescribably awful continuous pain, which is quite out of proportion to the patient's state of physical well-being.

Timing of pain

The timing of abdominal pain includes the frequency and duration of intermittent pains and the time of day when they occur, as well as the overall duration of pain. Ulcer pain tends to be worse towards the end of the day, seldom occurs before breakfast and does not always wake the patient at 2.00 a.m., as is usually thought. The pain of biliary colic is typically episodic and and unpredictable, with varying periods of complete freedom between attacks. Continuous pain for weeks or months in a patient not obviously dying of pancreatic or disseminated peritoneal cancer is usually functional. Pain which wakes the patient from sleep usually indicates organic disease but may also occur in functional problems.

Factors which modify pain

Modifying factors are of great help in diagnosis. Enquiry should routinely be made of the relationship of pain to meals, bowel actions and the passage of flatus, sexual intercourse, exertion and menstruation.

Most doctors ask about the relationship of any abdominal pain to *eating particular foods,* but there is little proof that such questions are discriminatory. For example, any type of abdominal pain, including functional abdominal pain, may be made worse by fatty or highly spiced foods. Fatty foods do not cause dyspepsia in patients with gallstones any more often than in normal people, or in patients with hiatus hernias or peptic ulcers.

Fat-induced dyspepsia does not suggest gallstones

It is rare to see a patient with an *allergy to a specific food.* This is usually recognised promptly by the patient as the food always gives rise to colicky abdominal pain and diarrhoea. Dietary cripples who have progressively pruned their diet to a few bland items almost always have a severe and irreversible alimentary neurosis. Attempts to broaden their diet almost always fail and are a waste of effort. I do not accept 'food intolerance' as a cause of multiple non-specific abdominal symptoms and general malaise and never prescribe elimination diets for these patients (see Chapter 14).

Patients with allergy to a specific food are rare

Apart from producing pain by allergic mechanisms some specific foods may cause abdominal pain. Lactose ingestion in lactase-deficient subjects may cause colicky abdominal pain and diarrhoea. It is, however, very uncommon for adults to present in this way, because symptomatic hypolactasics avoid lactose, though they are often not aware of the reason; they simply state that they 'don't like milk'. It is most unwise to ascribe abdominal pain or diarrhoea to hypolactasia until all other possible causes have been ruled out.

It is most unwise to ascribe abdominal pain or diarrhoea to hypolactasia

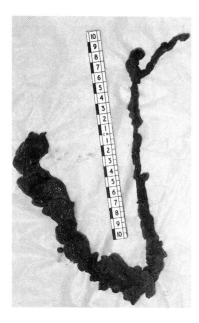

Fig. 6.1   An Australian nurse's stool: a vivid demonstration of colonic spasm!

Relief by defaecation and passage of flatus suggests colonic pain

---

Colonic pain may be felt anywhere in the abdomen and referred to bizarre extra-abdominal sites

---

Beware diagnosing functional pain coming on in later life

Alcohol may be related to pain; binge drinkers commonly have dyspepsia, and acute exacerbations of alcoholic chronic pancreatitis usually occur about 36 hours after a binge. Alcohol often immediately exacerbates peptic ulcer pain and the pain of the much rarer intestinal lymphomas. It may also exacerbate pain associated with colonic spasm, which is frequently associated with diarrhoea, usually six to twelve hours after the alcohol. Alcoholics tend to suffer not only from dyspepsia but also from diarrhoea.

Patients with coeliac disease occasionally report colicky abdominal pain following inadvertent gluten ingestion, but the psychological overlay is often enormous.

The *relationship of pain to meals,* regardless of their content, is of much more help. Symptoms experienced on an empty stomach suggest peptic ulceration, but give no indication as to the site. Relief by food suggests a duodenal ulcer and exacerbation by food, a gastric ulcer or gastric cancer. These relationships, however, are by no means invariable. Colonic pain is often felt in the epigastrium and may be related to feeding. The pain of intestinal angina is periumbilical, intense, crushing and steady. It comes on during each meal and may last for several hours; it is often relieved by nitrates. Diarrhoea and malabsorption may occur in patients with longstanding intestinal angina. The disease tends to progress over weeks or months to a fatal small bowel infarction, unless treated by vascular reconstruction.

The *relationship of pain to bowel actions and flatus* is very important and frequently not sought. Relief by bowel actions is very suggestive of a colonic origin for the pain. Relief is often only temporary and patients will often deny relief because the pain returns later. Colonic pain can be felt anywhere in the abdomen and is often associated with disordered bowel habit with the irregular passage of irregularly sized and shaped stools - at times like toothpaste, at times normal and at times like rabbit pellets (Fig. 6.1). A change in the pain may occur with constipation or diarrhoea and it may well have been made worse during a previous barium enema or sigmoidoscopy. If the pain is of long standing, or started in early life, it is almost certainly functional. However, one should beware the diagnosis of functional abdominal pain when a patient presents with a recent onset of pain, particularly above middle life. Functional abdominal pain does occur in older people, but the proportion of patients with underlying organic disease is high.

Musculoskeletal causes should be suspected if the pain is

exacerbated by excercise and relieved by rest, but many organic and functional abdominal pains show the same relation. Pain and tenderness which are still present or aggravated when the abdominal muscles are tensed (by getting the lying patient to lift the head and shoulders off the pillow with the arms folded) originates in the anterior abdominal wall.

Episodes of pain closely related to *menstruation* suggest endometriosis or pelvic inflammatory disease. Most abdominal pains are worsened premenstrually in those prone to premenstrual tension. The pelvic organs have for years borne the brunt of surgical attempts to cure functional abdominal pain and care is therefore needed to avoid unnecessary surgery.

If the predominant complaint is *belching* or excessive *rectal flatus without pain* the cause is almost always functional (see Chapter 17). It is often difficult to convince the patient of this diagnosis. Furthermore, since the acrophagy is often unconscious it can be even more difficult to cure. Abdominal distension and bloating, coming on rapidly over 10 minutes or so and usually in women, is a common but poorly recognised symptom of functional abdominal disease. The 'distension' is due to proptosis caused by arching of the back and by diaphragmatic descent, with relaxation of the anterior abdominal muscles. It is not due to fluid, acute obesity, constipation, swelling of the internal organs or rapid fermentation producing vast quantities of gas. Patients should be reassured. Sympathetic explanation is the only treatment.

Abdominal bloating - 'proptosis' - is a common functional symptom

Functional bowel disorders in perspective

Overall a wide variety of abdominal symptoms suggest functional abdominal disease, particularly if accompanied by graphic or bizarre descriptions, psychiatric disturbance or a long history.

Functional disorders account for about half the abdominal pain seen by all doctors, a rather greater proportion of those seen in a gastroenterology clinic, and almost all of those with abdominal pain lasting for years. A positive clinical diagnosis should usually be possible from a careful history. A limited number of investigations should be performed to exclude local organic disease; they are often required for the reassurance of both patient and doctor.

Many clinicians will diagnose functional abdominal symptoms only after meticulous investigation. This error of management is usually the result of impatient consultation and

The patient gets increasingly
frustrated by normal test results
despite continuing symptoms

a lack of clinical knowledge. Such mismanagement merely sustains the disorder, because the patient recognises the failure of the doctor to grasp the problem. The patient gets increasingly frustrated by a succession of normal test results, despite continuing symptoms.

Emotional or psychiatric disturbance is frequently denied at the initial and even subsequent interviews. Physicians should learn from psychiatrists and be prepared to spend time at several visits exploring emotional factors. Many patients with functional abdominal symptoms respond to antidepressant medication, though not obviously depressed in the classic sense. Careful establishment of rapport - which takes time - is sometimes necessary before the patient will admit depressive symptoms, such as lack of energy and drive, deteriorating concentration and memory, disordered sleep, persistent tiredness on waking, irritability, apathy, crying or a desire to cry, and ultimately suicidal thoughts.

Functional abdominal symptoms are surprisingly common in the general population. About 20% of the apparently normal British population have abdominal pain more than six times a year, and about 30% in all have symptoms generally recognised as functional. Fortunately, most of these patients do not bother to consult a doctor about their symptoms!

ABNORMALITIES ON EXAMINATION

Since the differential diagnosis of abdominal pain is so wide the potential findings on examination are correspondingly wide. A general physical examination, as well as a local abdominal examination with sigmoidoscopy, are usually required.

The following account is restricted to the positive features of functional abdominal disorders. The general aspect, body habitus and dress of the patient may arouse suspicion of depression, obsessionality or an attention-seeking personality. Either general examination is normal or the abnormalities discovered are irrelevant. Occasionally a patient worried by the possibility of dire disease in an embarassing area presents with abdominal pain and it may take time to get at the real problem. Abnormal findings, apart from tenderness, often over the colon, are conspicuous by their absence. Tenderness may occur over any part of the colon, particularly the sigmoid, though this area is palpable and somewhat tender in many normal people. Rectal examination should be normal.

Proctoscopy and sigmoidoscopy reveal a normal rectal mucosa. The rectum may be spastic and passage of the instrument or insufflation of air around the rectosigmoid junction may reproduce the pain of which the patient complains. This is not specific for functional colonic pain, but is highly suspicious.

It is important to be thorough and painstaking in physical examination, particularly if functional disease is suspected, because limited investigations only will be performed and misdiagnosis can occur.

INVESTIGATIONS

Once a functional bowel problem becomes the principal diagnosis, a planned limited investigation should be performed.

Screening tests

BLOOD COUNT AND ESR. A full blood count with measurement of the MCV should be performed to assess the likelihood particularly of iron deficiency, suggesting a bleeding lesion in the gut (low MCV), or B12 and folate deficiency, suggesting malabsorption of these vitamins (high MCV). Abnormal results at this stage require the doctor to reconsider the diagnosis or to admit the possibility of coexisting asymptomatic organic disease. A normal ESR is often taken as reassuring, but even extensive Crohn's disease or gastrointestinal cancer can both occur with a normal ESR. The reverse side of the coin is rather more reliable, though not absolutely so: a raised ESR suggests organic disease somewhere.

LIVER FUNCTION TESTS, ELECTROLYTES AND UREA. A raised alkaline phosphatase in patients with episodic abdominal pain suggests biliary disease or hepatic malignancy. If the alkaline phosphatase is of liver origin rather than from bone (confirmed by other abnormal liver enzymes, heat stability, or electrophoresis of the phosphatase) liver ultrasound and biopsy may be needed.

A low serum albumin concentration suggests organic disease, either of the manufacturing site in the liver or of the gut, due to excessive losses of plasma proteins - so-called 'protein-losing enteropathy'. This may occur with very many diseases of the gut, including colitis, Crohn's disease or gastrointestinal cancer.

Table 6.3 Investigation of persistent abdominal pain

Screening
Blood count and ESR
Liver biochemistry
Electrolytes and urea

Definitive
Barium meal and follow-
    through
Barium enema
Oral cholecystogram
Gastroscopy
Colonoscopy
Balloon distension studies

A low plasma potassium concentration suggests significant electrolyte losses, which would justify further investigation.

Definitive tests

RADIOLOGY. Radiological investigations should be ordered only after careful consideration. It is common for patients with functional abdominal symptoms to accumulate enormous exposure to X-rays in several different hospitals. Previously normal radiological investigation should not be unnecessarily repeated. Review of the films by clinician and radiologist together is very helpful.

Depending on the organic conditions within the differential diagnosis for an individual patient, a barium investigation may be required. Beware the clinician who orders for a patient a barium meal, followed by a small bowel follow-through and a barium enema: he is either considering Crohn's disease or does not understand the patient's symptoms. In the latter case the patient almost certainly has functional abdominal problems. Additional dangers in ordering too many investigations include the possibility of receiving irrelevant or even false information: some radiologists are notorious for seeing ulcers everywhere!

Cholecystography is vastly over-used. Gallstones cause biliary colic, jaundice or pancreatitis and are not responsible for dyspepsia or vague upper abdominal discomfort. The danger is that incidental gallstones will be found - and asymptomatic gallstones are extremely common in the uncomplaining population - and be blamed for the patient's symptoms. It is very vexing for both patient and doctor to remove the gallbladder, complete with stones, without curing the symptoms. The decision about the use of radiology in patients with abdominal pain should be left to a

Fig. 6.2 The equipment for balloon distension and the balloon in situ.

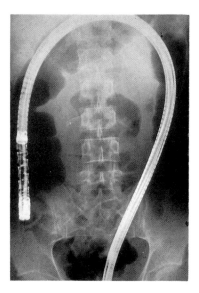

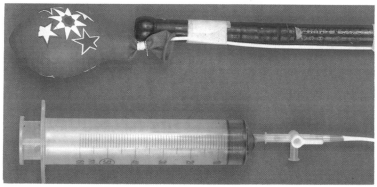

gastroenterologist, preferably one with some interest in functional abdominal disorders.

ENDOSCOPY. Similar considerations apply to endoscopy as to radiology. One great advantage of endoscopy is the lowering of the patient's guard by the intravenous diazepam used for sedation, allowing a closer approach to any underlying emotional problems. Selected endoscopy may be indicated to rule out specific organic problems, but all indiscriminate investigation is to be discouraged.

Research

In selected patients, balloon distension of the bowel (Fig. 6.2), performed in a specialist unit, may be of value. This is particularly the case in chronic sufferers from abdominal pain, who have consulted many doctors. The technique involves distending the colon, using a balloon attached to a colonoscope introduced per rectum, or distending the oesophagus and small bowel with a balloon introduced by mouth. The idea is to see whether distension will reproduce the patient's pain. Clearly distension of the bowel in anyone will produce pain. The key in this situation is the reproduction of the pain of which the patient complains. This demonstration frequently allows the patient to accept that the doctors know the cause of the pain (ascribed to a tender or spastic bowel), encouraging the patient to discontinue the search for a non-existent organic disorder.

MANAGEMENT

There is often no cure for functional abdominal symptoms of long standing. A sympathetic approach, however, is very important. The patient must feel that the practitioner believes that the patient has real abdominal symptoms and understands the mechanism of their production. This alone is often a great relief.

A detailed explanation with simple analogies, for instance to cramp in the leg muscles or 'asthma of the bowels', often brings a flash of understanding (albeit spurious) and relief of worry. Reassurance that the condition, whilst uncomfortable and a nuisance, is not dangerous, should not be treated by operation and has no complications, goes a long way to help the patient come to terms with the problem. An underlying fear of cancer is common; allaying this fear frequently also helps.

There is often no cure for functional abdominal pain of long standing

Table 6.4 Management of persistent abdominal pain

Sympathetic, thorough
    approach
Explanation
Treatment of stress or
    depression
High-fibre diet
Antispasmodics
Psychiatric help

Stress factors and underlying depression should be sought and treated. Antidepressants - amitriptyline 25-100 mg at night, mianserin 30-60 mg at night or imipramine 25-100 mg per day in divided doses - may be of value even in those who are not classically depressed. Bran, or any other bulk agent, may be useful, and a trial of a high-residue, and sometimes a low-residue, diet can be made. The response is rather unpredictable. A balanced intake of nutrients should, however, be encouraged.

Colonic antispasmodics before meals may help: mebeverine 135-270 mg three times daily given 20 minutes before meals, peppermint oil one or two capsules three times a day, or dicyclomine 10-20 mg three times daily.

A small proportion of patients are a terrible problem, particularly with unresponsive chronic pain. It may require all a physician's fortitude to forbear to operate for some spurious reason. The assistance of an interested psychiatrist may be of great value.

FURTHER READING

Dawson AM (1981) Abdominal symptoms. Med Int 12: 579-524.

Harvey RF, Salih SY, Read AE (1983) Organic and functional disorders in 2000 gastroenterology outpatients. Lancet 1: 632-634.

Lennard-Jones JE (1983) Functional gastrointestinal disorders. N Engl J Med 308: 431-435.

Pearson DJ, Rix KJB, Bentley SJ (1983) Food allergy: how much in the mind? Lancet 1: 1259-1261.

Review Article (1983) Irritable bowel syndrome and its treatment. Drug Ther Bull 21: 37-39.

Swarbrick ET, Bah L, Hegarty JE, Williams CB, Dawson AM (1980) Site of pain from the irritable bowel. Lancet 2: 443-446.

Thompson WG, Heaton KW (1980) Functional bowel disorders in apparently healthy people. Gastroenterology 79: 283-288.

Doctor, I've got terrible stomach ache ⁷

The patient with a severe acute abdominal pain usually has some form of organic disease. Consultation is usually as an emergency, often out of normal working hours, when the doctor may be rushed or exhausted.

However, a careful history and examination will often be rewarded by a correct clinical diagnosis, soon confirmed by hospital investigation or surgical exploration.

What are the common diagnoses? Acute appendicitis remains the most common cause of severe stomach pain in those admitted to hospital. Viral gastroenteritis and food poisoning, together with non-specific abdominal pain that remains undiagnosed and simply gets better of its own accord, must be seen much more frequently in general practice. Acute cholecystitis and acute diverticular disease are now more common than perforated peptic ulcer, while there is a steady increase in the number of patients with ruptured aneurysm and mesenteric ischaemia as a result of the increased incidence of atheroma and an ageing population. Renal calculi and small bowel adhesive obstruction are also on the increase and are among the common causes of sudden severe stomach ache.

> Consultation is usually an emergency but a careful history and examination will often be rewarded by a correct diagnosis

Table 7.1 Causes of severe abdominal pain

Infections/inflammation
Mechanical obstruction
Perforation
Vascular obstruction
Rupture and haemorrhage
Medical causes
'Catches'

DIFFERENTIAL DIAGNOSIS

The causes of severe abdominal pain can be divided into seven groups (Table 7.1).

Infection and inflammation

The first and largest group is infection or inflammation of one of the intra-abdominal organs ('the itises'). This group includes acute appendicitis, acute cholecystitis, acute pancreatitis, acute salpingitis, acute ileitis, acute diverticulitis, acute cystitis, acute pyelonephritis and acute gastroenteritis. These conditions are accompanied by a persistent aching pain

> Inflammation or infection of one of the abdominal organs is the commonest cause of sudden abdominal pain

of gradual onset and often produce fever and leucocytosis. Discomfort is usually felt over the anatomical site of the inflamed viscus.

Obstruction

The pain of obstruction is classically a colic

The pain of obstruction is brought about by blockage of a hollow tube, and made worse by the efforts of that tube to overcome the block. Small or large bowel obstruction, renal calculi and gallstones are the common causes of obstructive pain. This is classically a 'colic', with periods of relief or near-relief punctuated by episodes of severe pain which are often accompanied by agonised 'rolling about', sweating and vomiting.

Perforation

Perforation produces sudden severe stomach pain

Perforation of any intra-abdominal hollow viscus produces sudden severe stomach pain which is usually followed by signs of generalised peritonitis and shock. Peptic ulceration, acute appendicitis, acute diverticulitis and acute cholecystitis may all lead to perforation, which may also occur at or above sites of obstruction or result from intraluminal foreign bodies perforating the bowel wall. Perforation of the bowel may also be caused by endoscopic instrumentation or severe abdominal trauma.

Vascular obstruction

Strangulation, ischaemia or even frank gangrene can affect a number of organs within the intra-abdominal cavity. These changes are accompanied by severe abdominal pain and shock similar to that found after perforation. Small bowel ischaemia from strangulation, thrombosis, embolus, volvulus, intussusception or mesenteric damage is much more common than its large bowel equivalent. Gangrene of the appendix or gallbladder may follow infection. Fibroids and ovarian cysts may degenerate or twist, so becoming ischaemic and painful.

Visceral ischaemia can produce severe pain with little or no physical signs. Any patient who seems in agony but is found to have a soft abdomen must be suspected of having an ischaemic viscus: ischaemic pain is often so severe that, unlike almost any other abdominal pain, it is not relieved by intravenous narcotics.

Rupture and haemorrhage

Any intra-abdominal organ may rupture and bleed with signs of hypovolaemia accompanying the development of stomach pain. Ectopic pregnancy, ovarian cysts and even the pregnant uterus may rupture and bleed in this way; while relatively trivial trauma to a pathologically abnormal spleen or liver may produce immediate or delayed rupture with severe blood loss and pain. The kidneys, bladder and pancreas, in addition to the liver and spleen, are commonly damaged in severe road accidents when signs of hypovolaemia again suggest the cause of abdominal pain.

> Any abdominal organ may rupture and bleed with signs of hypovolaemia and stomach pain

Finally, a number of patients who have harboured a completely asymptomatic and unsuspected abdominal aneurysm may present for the first time with rupture, abdominal pain and shock. This diagnosis must be carefully excluded in any patient with a known aneurysm who develops sudden pain in the abdomen or back. Occasionally a leaking aneurysm masquerades as a more common condition, such as ureteric colic, backache, gastrointestinal bleeding or mesenteric ischaemia, but the diagnosis usually becomes clear as shock develops with increasing abdominal tenderness, swelling, bruising or a mass.

Free blood in the abdominal cavity can cause a variable amount of pain which may be referred to the shoulder tip if blood comes in contact with the diaphragm. The degree of associated peritonism on palpation is also extremely variable, ranging from marked to minimal.

Medical conditions

A number of conditions not requiring surgery may produce pain in the abdomen. Basal pneumonia, myocardial infarction, pericarditis and pulmonary embolus have all been misdiagnosed as an acute abdomen and may be confidently diagnosed only by careful examination and the application of specialised tests.

Viral diseases like Coxsackie infections, infectious mononucleosis, herpes zoster and infectious hepatitis may also create diagnostic difficulty, but abdominal signs are usually minimal or absent in these conditions. Early presumptive diagnosis must await confirmatory serological tests.

Diabetics occasionally experience abdominal pain and vomiting during hyperglycaemic ketoacidosis. Rare conditions like porphyria, lead poisoning, sickle cell disease and tabes dorsalis need consideration only when other commoner causes of abdominal pain have been excluded.

Catches

Finally, a few catches or diagnostic pitfalls must not be forgotten. Referred stomach pain from torsion of the testis or a strangulated hernia must be excluded by the relevant examination. Similarly spinal pain with abdominal referral must also be considered in the absence of other pathology.

Severe acute abdominal pain is rarely of psychological origin; this diagnosis should be considered only if pethidine addiction or Munchausen's syndrome is suspected. The pethidine addict may have tell-tale venepuncture marks in his antecubital fossa and other sites, whilst the Munchausen often has multiple abdominal scars from procedures which, with hindsight, may not have been strictly necessary.

Dysmenorrhoea, constipation, mesenteric adenitis, Mittelschmerz and the irritable bowel syndrome may all produce mild abdominal pain but can be confirmed as the cause of pain only when all other possibilities have been excluded. Conditions within the abdominal wall such as a spontaneous inferior epigastric haematoma may also occasionally give rise to diagnostic difficulty.

Severe acute abdominal pain is rarely of psychological origin

---

CLUES FROM THE HISTORY

As in most conditions a carefully taken history is very important in correctly diagnosing the cause of stomach ache (Table 7.2).

Pain

If the patient recalls the precise moment of onset of the pain then perforation, vascular obstruction or rupture with haemorrhage are the most likely pathological processes. The 'itises' and mechanical obstructions usually start gradually and build up over a period to more severe pain.

The duration of the pain may also be helpful. Pains of a few minutes' duration need reassessment unless they are obviously pathological or are accompanied by shock. Beware the golden period in patients with perforation: after severe initial stomach ache the pain can disappear before generalised peritonitis,

Table 7.2   History of pain in patients with severe abdominal pain

Onset
Sudden: perforation
           vascular obstruction
           haemorrhage or rupture
Gradual: inflammation/infection
           mechanical obstruction
           many 'medical' causes

Duration
Less than 1 hour: reassess unless vascular problem or
                     perforation
More than 6 hours: inflammation
                     obstruction
                     perforation
Months or years: usually no pathological cause found

Site
See Fig. 7.1

Radiation
See Fig. 7.2

Character
See Fig. 7.3

Aggravating and relieving factors
Staying still: peritonitis
Rolling around: colic

Severity
Very severe: gangrene of an organ
Mild: may simply indicate a stoical patient

Shifting nature
Appendicitis
Perforated ulcer

Associated symptoms
See Table 7.3

shock and septicaemia develop. Pain lasting for more than six hours is usually of pathological significance. At the other end of the scale stomach ache that has been present in some form for many years is often difficult to diagnose unless it is associated with a sudden severe exacerbation.

The site of pain within the abdomen is very helpful if it can be satisfactorily localised by the patient. Typical situations are shown in Fig. 7.1. At the same time any site of referral or radiation must also be carefully elicited (Fig. 7.2) and any change in position of the pain noted. The pain of appendicitis, for instance, starts centrally and moves to the right iliac fossa.

Next the type or character of the pain should be sought. There are two main forms of abdominal pain. The first is the pain of peritonitis which is a continuous persistent gnawing ache made worse by movement, coughing, laughing or straining. Peritoneal pain is minimised by the patient keeping absolutely still. The second pain is colic produced by mechanical obstruction. True colic comes only from the intestine and consists of short episodes of pain punctuated by periods of complete relief. The length of the gaps between pain gives some idea of the level of intestine which is affected.

> There are two main forms of abdominal pain: peritonitis and colic

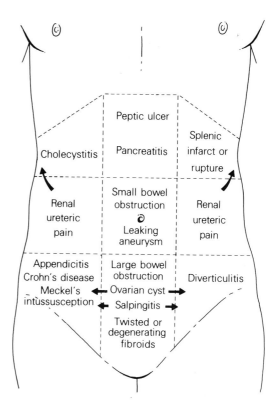

Fig. 7.1   Primary sites of stomach ache.

Intervals of 10 to 15 seconds between the pain are found with high small bowel obstruction, intervals of up to one to two minutes in ileal disease and intervals as long as 5 to 10 minutes in large bowel obstruction. Both biliary and ureteric calculus obstruction produce 'colic', but this differs from true colic in that a constant background pain is always present, although episodes of even more severe pain occur at regular intervals. The frequency and nature of these pains are summarised in Fig. 7.3. Patients with a ruptured aortic aneurysm often report a 'tearing pain' and patients with ischaemic small bowel have very severe and shocking pain often out of proportion to their signs. However, all other descriptions of pain tend to be more graphic than helpful, depending more upon the descriptive ability and sensitivity of the patients than their abdominal condition.

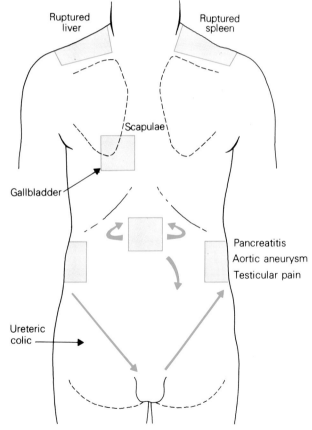

Fig. 7.2   Sites of referred pain.

Table 7.3 Checklist for symptoms associated with severe abdominal pain

Upper gastrointestinal
Vomiting
Nausea
Loss of appetite
Loss of weight
Previous indigestion
Stool colour
Urine colour
White medicine
Barium meal, endoscopy, etc.
Reflux
Waterbrash
Exotic meals

Lower gastrointestinal
Diarrhoea
Constipation (absolute)
Mucus
Blood per rectum
Slime

Genitourinary
Dysuria
Frequency
Haematuria

Menstrual
Date of last period
Number of days in last period
Number of days between
   periods
Intermenstrual bleeding
Vaginal discharge
Symptoms of pregnancy

Trauma

Previous operations

Previous illnesses

Drugs

Allergies

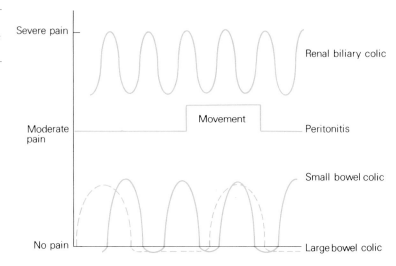

Fig. 7.3   The characteristics of abdominal pains.

Aggravating and relieving factors have already been described. Patients with peritonitis lie still and the pain is made worse by any form of movement or abdominal straining, while patients with colic roll around and cannot find a comfortable spot. The pain of an acute abdomen is rarely relieved by mild analgesia.

Associated symptoms (Table 7.3)

Symptoms of nausea and vomiting and abnormality of appetite must always be noted since all major intra-abdominal pathology is associated with a disturbance of upper gastrointestinal function. Gastroenteritis, pelvic or retro-ileal appendicitis, regional ileitis and carcinoma of the rectum all increase the frequency of bowel action. Absolute constipation is one of the main features of complete large bowel obstruction. Previous passage of blood, mucus and slime per rectum may give further support to a large bowel pathology as the cause of pain.

A past history of indigestion may suggest peptic ulceration, cholecystitis or hiatus hernia and lead to additional questions on the relationship of pain to food, the types of food producing the pain and previous investigations and medications for dyspepsia. If gallstones are suspected the patient should always be asked if the urine or stool changed colour during or after previous episodes of pain. A history of reflux or waterbrash may again point to a diagnosis of hiatus hernia or peptic ulceration. Weight loss is associated with a number of intra-abdominal conditions, especially intra-abdominal malignancy, gastric ulceration, Crohn's disease and chronic mesenteric arterial insufficiency. If a diagnosis of gastroenteritis or food poisoning is suspected in a patient complaining of colicky abdominal pain with diarrhoea and vomiting, the story of an unusual meal or a visit to an exotic restaurant may provide additional support for the diagnosis.

A history of haematuria, urinary frequency or dysuria may suggest that a calculus or urinary tract infection is the cause of pain, whereas cough, haemoptysis, green sputum, pain on respiration or shortness of breath suggest pneumonia, pulmonary embolism or pleurisy. Any story of preceding trauma, even if it is apparently trivial, may be the only clue to a diagnosis of intra-abdominal haemorrhage from damage to the spleen, liver or other organs.

Women with stomach ache should always be questioned about their periods and obstetric history since the important diagnosis of ectopic pregnancy can be clinched by an appropriate story of a missing or delayed period. Ectopic pregnancy has been described at any interval after the last period and is not excluded simply because of recent vaginal blood loss that the patient thought was menstrual. Unfortunately, patients with salpingitis rarely give a history of profuse purulent vaginal discharge which is more commonly associated with monilial vaginitis. The presence of a coil should alert the doctor to the possibility of pelvic inflammatory disease. Sudden onset of mid-cycle pain of short duration suggests the diagnosis of a ruptured ovarian cyst or Mittelschmerz. Other complications of ovarian cysts or fibroids will seldom be suspected from the history and must be detected by the appropriate findings on physical examination.

In all patients with stomach ache a past history of similar pains must be sought. Relevant past operations and illnesses must be fully documented since these may have important bearing on the present pain. Drugs and allergies should also be noted before physical examination is carried out.

> Women with stomach pains should be asked about menstrual and obstetric history

ABNORMALITIES ON EXAMINATION

General examination

The patient is examined for evidence of dehydration, anaemia, tachycardia, fever and hypotension. The tongue may be furred and the breath foetid in acute gastrointestinal disease such as appendicitis. All the major lymph node groups should be palpated and the chest examined for signs of pleurisy, pneumonia and cardiac abnormality.

Abdominal examination

Abdominal examination must be conducted in a good light with the patient fully undressed

This must be conducted in a good light with the patient fully undressed from the nipples to the mid-thigh so that the groins and genitalia are exposed. The patient should lie flat and relaxed on a couch or a bed. The time honoured routine of inspection, palpation, percussion and auscultation is then followed.

INSPECTION. Scars, lumps, distension and abdominal movement with respiration are all noted. Scars may indicate an adhesive obstruction while lumps may be tumours, hernias, obstructed organs, inflammatory masses, abscesses or haematomas within the abdomen or its wall. The abdomen is centrally distended in patients with small bowel obstruction and distended around the periphery in large bowel obstruction. Distension is also found with large ovarian cysts, fibroids, pancreatic pseudocysts, pregnancy and ascites. Peritonitis is associated with reduced movement of the abdominal wall, since this minimises the pain. At a late stage, patients with generalised peritonitis develop abdominal swelling as vast quantities of fluid exude into the peritoneal cavity and peristalsis ceases.

PALPATION AND PERCUSSION. This is gently and systematically carried out with the flat of the hand around the whole abdomen. Initially, tenderness is looked for on light palpation, indicating sites of local pathology; then deep palpation reveals guarding (involuntary muscle contraction) at sites of local peritonitis. The totally rigid abdomen is usually instantly obvious and precludes any attempt at deep palpation. Percussion is also a good method of confirming rebound tenderness and should be carried out in any areas of guarding.

Rigidity, guarding and rebound indicate significant local peritonitis

The presence of rigidity, guarding and rebound all indicate significant local peritonitis.

Masses observed on inspection must be carefully reassessed by palpation and percussion. A number of lumps that were not obvious on inspection will be detected by the examining hand and the detection of any lump is of extreme diagnostic importance. Inflammatory masses can occur in association with the gallbladder, appendix, pancreas, sigmoid colon and uterine (fallopian) tubes. Large ovarian cysts and fibroids may be palpable above the pelvic brim and must be distinguished from the enlarged bladder of urinary retention. A large central expansile pulsatile mass is diagnostic of an abdominal aortic aneurysm. Colonic carcinoma and diverticular masses are often impalpable in patients with obstruction.

Percussion, in addition to showing localised areas of rebound tenderness, may distinguish free fluid within the abdomen.

Rectal and vaginal examination should be carefully performed in all patients with a severe stomach ache. Rectal, ovarian and uterine tumours are often more easily detected when rectal and vaginal examination are combined with abdominal examination as a bimanual. The genitalia and hernial orifices must also routinely be palpated at the beginning or end of any abdominal examination to avoid missing significant pathology on cursory abdominal examination.

AUSCULTATION. Ascultation is usually used in the abdomen to detect the presence or absence of bowel sounds. Absent bowel sounds indicate the presence of an ileus or peritonitis, while frequent amphoteric bowel sounds are heard in patients with large bowel obstruction. The presence of an abdominal bruit rarely signifies an aortic aneurysm unless complicated by an aortocaval fistula, but it is sometimes found in patients with mesenteric ischaemia; more commonly an abdominal bruit is due to incidental aorto-iliac atheroma.

Summary

In the absence of a definite diagnosis at the end of the history and examination the general practitioner has to place the patient in one of three categories:

1. The patient has an acute problem within the abdomen which requires transfer to hospital for a surgical opinion.

2. The patient has no serious intra-abdominal pathology. The patient's condition will settle with simple medication or no treatment at all while he remains at home.

3. The patient could have serious pathology. This patient must be re-examined in a few hours time or transferred to hospital for further observation.

If the first or last options are followed it is often helpful to discuss the case history directly with the duty surgical registrar at the local hospital before any analgesia is administered. Patients in the first group who are in severe pain should be given suitable analgesia before transfer to hospital since obvious peritonitis is rarely masked by opiates.

INVESTIGATIONS

There are few investigations, apart from taking the temperature, which can be performed on patients with severe stomach ache outside hospital. If a confident diagnosis of gastroenteritis or urinary tract infection is made, appropriate samples should be sent to a bacteriology laboratory before antibiotic treatment, if indicated, is commenced.

Most other investigations should be carried out in hospital and will be dictated by either the differential or working diagnosis obtained from the history and examination.

Routine urine testing with a dipstick for blood, sugar, protein and bile should be carried out on all patients attending hospital, and may provide useful information in patients with cholecystitis, renal colic or diabetes. Many patients with a confident diagnosis of acute appendicitis require little in the way of investigation. However, most anaesthetists require a haemoglobin estimation before operation and the opportunity can be taken to carry out a white cell count which, if raised, may add further support to the diagnosis of an acute inflammatory process. A sickle cell screening test is always necessary in patients of African origin before a general anaesthetic; very rarely abdominal pain may be due to a sickle cell crises.

The presence of free gas under the diaphragm on erect chest or abdominal X-ray (Fig. 7.4) provides useful confirmation of a perforated ulcer or perforation elsewhere within the gastrointestinal tract. This sign may, however, be absent in up to one-fifth of all patients with a perforation. Plain abdominal X-rays may also show up distended bowel with fluid levels in obstruction (Figs 7.5, 7.6), gallstones (Fig. 7.7), renal calculi (Fig. 7.8) and calcification outlining the wall of an abdominal aneurysm (Fig. 7.9). A pair of plain X-rays provide the most useful investigation for a patient with undiagnosed abdominal pain. However, abdominal X-rays reveal no abnormality at all in a number of serious conditions, and a normal X-ray must never override the clinical impression formed from the history

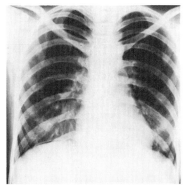

Fig. 7.4 Free gas under the right diaphragm, shown on an erect chest X-ray.

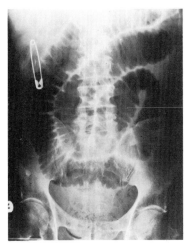

Fig. 7.5 Distended small bowel with the ladder pattern in small bowel obstruction.

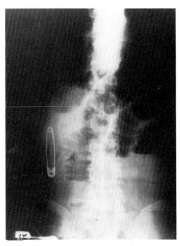

Fig. 7.6 Fluid levels in small bowel obstruction.

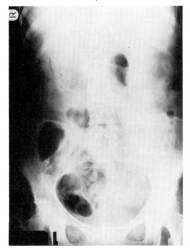

Fig. 7.7 Calcified gallstones in the right upper quadrant of the gallbladder, outlined by gas in the wall.

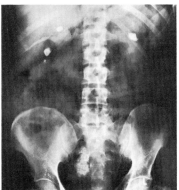

Fig. 7.8 An oval calculus in the lower right ureter, lying over the wing of the sacrum.

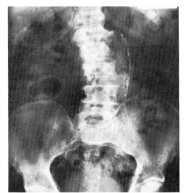

Fig. 7.9 An abdominal aortic aneurysm seen as a soft-tissue mass overlying the left psoas muscle with calcium in the wall.

and examination. A chest X-ray and ECC will exlude serious disease within the chest, while more sophisticated tests of lung and cardiac function may be carried out later if the diagnosis remains in doubt.

A serum amylase should be taken from all patients with sudden severe stomach ache if the diagnosis is in doubt as laparotomy is still better avoided in patients with acute pancreatitis. Confirmatory tests for acute pancreatitis include the serum calcium, ultrasound examination and CAT scan, and now even ERCP has been advocated.

Acute cholecystitis may be confirmed by ultrasonography or oral cholecystography in the 85% of patients whose gallstones are radiolucent.

Patients with possible renal or ureteric calculi should have urgent intravenous pyelography to confirm the diagnosis. Subsequent management will be affected by the degree of renal obstruction that is present on the pyelogram.

Patients thought to have non-perforating peptic ulceration of the stomach or duodenum may await endoscopy or barium studies, but a reasonable suspicion of perforation, even in the absence of free gas on plain film, should lead directly to laparotomy. Urgent contrast studies may be misleading and are not widely used to confirm perforation. Endoscopy is contraindicated if perforation is suspected, as the procedure may increase flow from the gut lumen to the peritoneum.

The diagnosis of small bowel obstruction can usually be made on the plain film. Small bowel radiographs are only required for subacute obstruction, especially if the diagnosis of Crohn's disease is suspected. All patients with suspected large bowel obstruction should have a sigmoidoscopy performed and, in contrast to the patients with small bowel obstruction, a barium enema examination is helpful. It will prevent unnecessary laparotomy in patients with pseudo-obstruction and ensure that the correct incision and approach is made for primary resection of an obstructing lesion (Figs 7.10, 7.11). Barium enema should not be performed when obstruction is accompanied by significant caecal tenderness or distension because of risk of perforation if operative decompression is delayed.

Clinical suspicion of salpingitis, ruptured ovarian cyst or ectopic pregnancy can be confirmed by laparoscopy, while a large twisted ovarian cyst or degenerating fibroid may be evident on ultrasound examination.

Abdominal aortic aneurysms can also be confirmed by ultrasound examination (which measures the diameter of the aorta), but if a CAT scanner is available this is capable of showing retroperitoneal clot and differentiating an acute expanding aneurysm from a small leak.

MANAGEMENT

Acute appendicitis

This should be treated by appendicectomy unless an appendix mass is present when delay for six to eight weeks is advisable.

Early surgery is still indicated if the mass is associated with peritonitis or an abscess. There is little or no place for conservative management of straightforward acute appendicitis by bed rest and antibiotics.

There is no place for conservative management of acute appendicitis

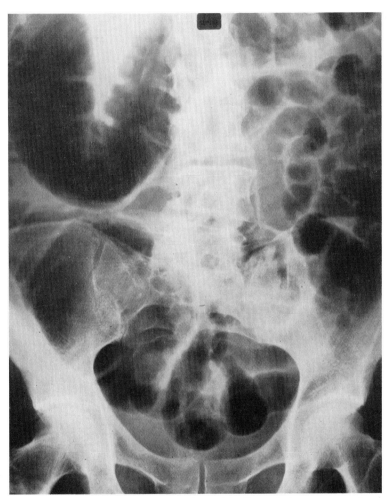

Fig. 7.10 Large bowel obstruction with distended caecum and right colon shown on a plain X-ray of the abdomen.

Acute cholecystitis

The standard initial managment is conservative, with bed rest, analgesia and, if indicated, antibiotics, nasogastric suction and intravenous fluids. The majority of patients settle with this regimen and, after confirmation of the diagnosis, elective

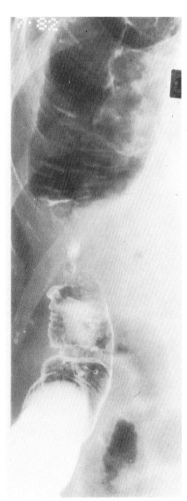

Fig. 7.11 A barium enema from the same patient as Fig. 7.10, showing an obstructive lesion consistent with a carcinoma in the descending colon.

cholecystectomy is performed six to eight weeks after the acute attack. Early surgery is indicated if signs of spreading peritonitis develop or the acute attack fails to settle with conservative measures. Recently a number of centres have advocated prompt diagnosis and early surgery. It is suggested that operations may be easier at this stage and the approach has the additional advantage that early surgery avoids the expense of a second admission to hospital. The results of random allocation to one of these two treatment policies are awaited.

Perforated peptic ulceration

Patients with a perforated ulcer should be given suitable analgesia and prepared for urgent laparotomy with nasogastric suction and intravenous fluids. Few if any patients should be treated conservatively since all the published studies show that early ulcer closure halves the mortality of medical treatment. Resuscitation should be abandoned in favour of surgery if improvement is not quickly obtained since some patients will improve only when the gastric contents are sucked out of the peritoneal cavity. Simple closure of the perforation is the treatment of choice in sick patients with heavy contamination but some form of definitive surgery may be carried out in fit patients, with a long history of indigestion. This avoids re-operation which may be required on up to half the patients treated by simple closure. This figure may, however, be reduced by the long-term use of the H_2-blockers cimetidine or ranitidine, which will prevent recurrence.

Acute pancreatitis

Sick patients with this condition require urgent resuscitation with intravenous fluids, colloid and blood. Fluid replacement should be monitored by a central venous pressure line, frequent haematocrit estimations and an indwelling urethral catheter. Patients should receive adequate analgesia and oxygen, if this is indicated by arterial blood gas analysis. Calcium replacement may also be required to avoid the development of tetany. The onset of renal or respiratory failure may require peritoneal dialysis or controlled ventilation. Peritoneal lavage may prove useful therapy for the pancreatitis itself, in addition to overcoming renal failure. Early hopes that glucagon or aprotinin would prove beneficial have not been borne out by the MRC trial. The place of laparotomy is also unclear.

Surgical drainage of the pancreas with decompression of the common bile duct may be superseded by peritoneal dialysis and ERCP with endoscopic sphincterotomy and removal of duct stones where indicated. The complications of pseudocyst or abscess formation must be treated by surgical drainage while, if the diagnosis of acute pancreatitis remains in doubt, laparotomy must be performed to exclude perforation or ischaemia of the bowel.

Small bowel obstruction

An obstructed or strangulated hernia must be suspected and carefully excluded in all patients with small bowel obstruction. If a tender irreducible lump is found at an appropriate site (usually the groin), in association with small bowel obstruction, this must be considered the likely cause, and urgent surgery carried out through an appropriately sited incision.

All other patients with undiagnosed small bowel obstruction must be considered potential candidates for laparotomy to prevent the development of unsuspected strangulation and gangrene of the obstructed loop. Exceptions to this management policy may, however, be made. Patients who are suspected of having postoperative adhesive obstruction may be treated conservatively with nasogastric suction and intravenous fluid replacement. If the pain, pulse rate and abdominal tenderness all settle rapidly, and further abdominal X-rays suggest that gas is passing on into the colon, this treatment may be maintained while spontaneous resolution of the obstruction occurs. Patients suspected of having Crohn's disease may await investigation with a small bowel meal (Fig. 7.12). Medical treatment with steroids or sulphasalazine may resolve the inflammation and avoid surgical resection. All other patients should proceed to early laparotomy after appropriate preoperative preparation to ensure their fitness for anaesthesia.

Large bowel obstruction

Early surgery for suspected large bowel obstruction is indicated if there is marked abdominal tenderness or gross caecal distension on the plain X-ray, when there is a real danger of perforation. Most patients may await barium enema confirmation of obstruction if rectal examination and sigmoidoscopy fail to provide a diagnosis. After appropriate fluid replacement and preoperative antibiotics (intravenous

Fig. 7.12 A long stricture in the terminal ileum (Kantor's string sign), consistent with Crohn's disease, revealed by a small bowel meal.

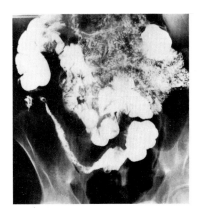

metronidazole) laparotomy can be carried out through an incision which will allow primary resection of the obstructing lesion (usually a carcinoma or diverticular disease). If primary anastomosis is undertaken a covering colostomy is advisable to prevent subsequent peritonitis if anastomotic dehiscence should occur. It is often preferable to avoid anastomosis by exteriorising the proximal bowel and either exteriorising the distal stump or closing it off as a blind-ended rectal stump (a Hartman's procedure) if it will not reach the abdominal wall. This makes a two-stage rather than a three-stage procedure with the benefit that the pathology is totally removed at the first stage, thus avoiding the risk of metastatic spread from tumour manipulation at the first laparotomy.

Diverticulitis

Localised tenderness over the sigmoid colon with or without a mass will usually respond to antibiotics. Metronidazole, gentamicin and possibly ampicillin are a highly effective combination. If there are signs of increasing local or developing generalised peritonitis, laparotomy and excisional surgery is the treatment of choice with exteriorisation of both bowel ends. The classical procedure of proximal colostomy and drainage is less successful than excisional surgery.

Salpingitis and urinary tract infection

These conditions require appropriate antibiotic treatment which may be started before culture results are available and then adjusted appropriately. A sulphonamide, trimethoprim, ampicillin or a cephalosporin may all be used as first-line treatment.

Ruptured or twisted ovarian cyst

Many ruptured follicular cysts presenting in mid-cycle with typical Mittelschmerz are best treated expectantly, but larger malignant ovarian cysts presenting with severe abdominal pain require laparotomy and excision. If the cysts are very large or appear carcinomatous oophorectomy is indicated. Bilateral oophorectomy and concomitant hysterectomy to remove sites of secondary spread is the treatment of choice in carcinoma of the ovary. If widespread malignancy is present maximal tumour debulking should be carried out with an added omentectomy before treatment with radiotherapy and cytotoxic drugs is begun.

Twisted or degenerating fibroid

This should be treated by local myomectomy or hysterectomy where appropriate.

Ruptured ectopic pregnancy

This diagnosis may be obvious if accompanied by severe shock. Emergency surgery with tubal excision is then usually necessary to preserve life. If, however, the onset is insidious and suspected only because of a forniceal mass or a positive pregnancy test, confirmation of the diagnosis by laparoscopy may lead to tubal conservation by a suitably experienced gynaecologist.

Leaking aortic aneurysm

After a quick initial assessment and cross-matching has been carried out patients are transferred to theatre with minimal resusciatation to avoid increasing the haematoma and to prevent re-bleeding. Aortic cross-clamping of the aneurysm neck should be carried out as rapidly as possible. Then, after adequate resuscitation, an appropriate prosthesis may be inlaid within the aneurysm sac. A minor controlled retroperitoneal bleed from an aortic aneurysm is easily misdiagnosed as a painful expanding aneurysm and will be diagnosed with certainty only by an emergency CAT scan.

Mesenteric infarction, volvulus and intussusception

The first two conditions require urgent laparotomy and bowel resection. Intussusception may be satisfactorily reduced at an early stage by barium enema but a careful watch must be kept on the patient to ensure that perforation or gangrene are not developing. If reduction fails or complications develop laparotomy and surgical reduction or resection is required.

Renal and ureteric calculi

Calculi may be treated expectantly unless there is a danger of a pyonephrosis or anuria developing with a stone obstructing a solitary kidney. Large stones which are unlikely to pass, together with stones producing persistent obstruction or symptoms, require surgical removal. Dormia basket extraction is useful in speeding the removal of small stones below the pelvic brim, whilst direct urethrolithotomy remains the treatment of choice for larger stones above this level. Ultrasonic dissolution of stones is not yet readily available or effective.

Abdominal trauma

Confirmation of intra-abdominal damage may be obtained by peritoneal lavage. Organ reconstruction or resection is dictated by the laparotomy findings. In children every attempt should be made to preserve splenic tissue to prevent the development of serious infection in the future.

Undiagnosed stomach ache

Patients in whom a diagnosis cannot be made should be managed expectantly while appropriate investigations are undertaken. Re-examination at regular intervals will show if an acute abdomen is developing. Laparotomy is then indicated. Blind laparotomy in patients with undiagnosed abdominal pain and minimal signs is rarely of benefit. Frequent reassessment remains the cornerstone of management, with laparotomy the final court of appeal.

FURTHER READING

Cox C (1978) Glucagon and aprotinin in the treatment of acute pancreatitis: MRC multicentre trial. Ann R Coll Surg Engl 60: 141-143.

McArthur P, Cuscheri A, Shields R, Sells RA (1975) Controlled clinical trial comparing early with interval cholecystectomy for acute cholecystitis. Proc R Soc Med 68: 32-36.

Mitchell A, Morris PJ (1982) Trends in management of acute cholecystitis. Br Med J 284: 27-30.

Shepherd JA (1975) Concise Surgery of the Acute Abdomen. Edinburgh: Churchill Livingstone.

Silen W (1979) Cope's Early Diagnosis of the Acute Abdomen. London: Oxford University Press.

Welch CE, Malt RA (1983) Abdominal surgery, parts 1 and 3. N Engl J Med 308: 624-632, 753-759.

Doctor, I've gone yellow

8

The appearance of yellow discoloration of the skin usually signifies the onset of jaundice, although mild degrees may be difficult to detect. Rarely, jaundice may be imitated by raised blood carotene levels from myxoedema or carrot juice 'health' diets, but true jaundice results from raised levels of bilirubin in the blood. A simple review of the pathophysiology is helpful in understanding the causes and differential diagnosis (Fig. 8.1). Bilirubin is a breakdown product of haem in red cells and is released into the blood stream as unconjugated bilirubin. In this form it is not water-soluble and is not excreted in urine, hence the term 'acholuric jaundice' (absence of bile from the urine) for the unconjugated causes of jaundice such as haemolysis. Once conjugated by liver enzymes, bilirubin becomes water-soluble and is excreted into bile. Disturbance of

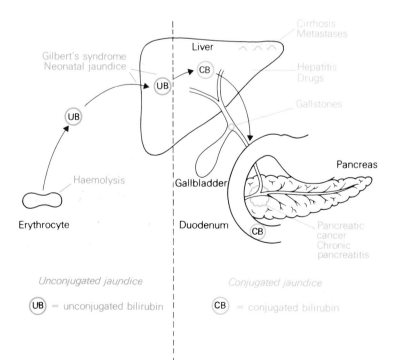

Fig. 8.1 The pathophysiology of jaundice.

biliary secretion, through either liver disease or mechanical blockage, will result in jaundice of the 'conjugated' type and excess bilirubin is excreted by the kidneys to produce the familiar dark urine.

DIFFERENTIAL DIAGNOSIS

The most important causes of 'unconjugated' jaundice are excessive haemolysis such as occurs in sickle cell disease or hereditary spherocytosis, and are not the result of any liver disease.

Unconjugated jaundice due to haemolysis is not the result of liver disease

Gilbert's syndrome should be specifically mentioned. Its cause, though not known precisely, is probably a mixture of low-grade haemolysis, impaired hepatic uptake and defective conjugation of unconjugated bilirubin, and it is an extremely common cause of mild unconjugated jaundice that affects about 1-2% of the population. It is entirely benign, but it is important to be aware of the condition in order to reassure the patient and his life insurance company that he has a normal liver. The jaundice is mild, often picked up on a routine biochemical profile, but may increase in intensity during fasting or intercurrent illness. Hence patients are often mistakenly thought to have viral hepatitis when they become mildly icteric during an attack of influenza. Remember that bilirubin is absent from the urine. The jaundice appears to subside in later life.

Gilbert's syndrome is entirely benign

The causes of conjugated jaundice all reflect liver or biliary disease. The commonest of these is viral hepatitis, an illness of increasing complexity for the virologist who identifies the causal agents, but still fairly straightforward for the clincian. Type A, formerly called infective hepatitis, has a short incubation period of about four to six weeks, is spread by the orofaecal route, and does not become chronic or cause cirrhosis. Type B ('Australia antigen'), formerly called serum hepatitis, has an incubation period of 50 to 60 days, may be spread both parenterally and non-parenterally, and carries a real risk of chronic infection and cirrhosis. Type non-A non-B is still a 'ragbag' diagnosis of exclusion but is the commonest type of post-transfusion hepatitis in the USA and UK now that donor blood is screened for hepatitis B. It is thought to produce chronic liver disease in some recipients. Glandular fever must not be forgotten as a cause of viral hepatitis; 90% of sufferers have disturbed liver function tests and a minority develop overt jaundice.

The diagnosis of viral hepatitis may be difficult in the elderly. In this age group particularly, the patient may be on a range of medications for other conditions and drug-induced jaundice must always be considered.

Jaundice may also be the presenting symptom of chronic liver disease, either chronic hepatitis or cirrhosis. Deaths from cirrhosis have doubled in the last decade, and this is solely the result of increasing alcohol consumption. At least 70% of cases of cirrhosis are directly attributable to alcohol. Other causes are given in Table 8.1 and include primary biliary cirrhosis and chronic hepatitis B infection.

Jaundice is the cardinal feature of extrahepatic biliary obstruction, most cases of which are due to either a gallstone impacted in the common bile duct or a carcinoma of the pancreas. Pancreatic cancer, because of its late presentation, has an appalling prognosis. Just occasionally a tumour in the head of the gland or arising in the papilla of Vater will be operable and curable because early jaundice draws attention to the diagnosis. The bile duct can be obstructed in its course through the pancreas by chronic pancreatitis, usually alcoholic. The differentiation between chronic pancreatitis and carcinoma may be difficult and this probably explains at least some long-term survivors from apparent carcinoma. Malignant disease may also cause jaundice through diffuse liver infiltration or through obstruction of the biliary tree, for instance by enlarged lymph nodes in the porta hepatis.

CLUES FROM THE HISTORY

It is usually possible to make a diagnosis or draw up a limited differential diagnosis on the basis of the history, leaving the examination and investigations to confirm this. The salient clues to be looked for in each condition are taken in turn.

Viral hepatitis

This diagnosis usually poses few problems in children and young adults. A history of exposure should be sought, bearing in mind the incubation period of six weeks to six months, including travel to endemic areas, blood transfusions and injections. Remember the risks of exposure at work for medical personnel and the greatly increased frequency of hepatitis B (and probably hepatitis A) infection in male homosexuals.

Drug-induced jaundice must not be overlooked, especially in the elderly

Jaundice may be the presenting symptom of chronic liver disease

Jaundice is the cardinal feature of extrahepatic biliary obstruction

Table 8.1   Some causes of cirrhosis

Alcohol
Hepatitis B
Primary biliary cirrhosis
'Lupoid' chronic hepatitis
Alpha-1-antitrypsin deficiency
Haemochromatosis
Wilson's disease
Cardiac cirrhosis
Secondary biliary cirrhosis
Drugs (e.g. oxyphenisatin)
Cryptogenic

Remember the greatly increased incidence of hepatitis in male homosexuals

A prodromal illness before the onset of jaundice includes anorexia or vomiting, and there may be a fleeting skin rash or arthritis, particularly in type B infection. Patients often lose their taste for smoking. After a prodrome of a few days to a week, the patient usually notices dark urine just before the jaundice becomes obvious. Parodoxically, as jaundice is established, the patient begins to feel better and starts to eat again. Itching may develop during this phase and jaundice usually subsides after about a fortnight. A little abdominal discomfort is usual but may occasionally be severe, resulting in emergency surgical admission and even inappropriate laparotomy, particularly in the early phase of viral hepatitis.

Diagnosis is more difficult in the elderly and in variants of acute viral hepatitis, such as relapsing hepatitis and prolonged cholestasis. In the latter the patient may remain profoundly jaundiced for several months, and here specialised imaging techniques are required to exclude mechanical obstruction.

Alcohol

The importance of considering alcohol as a cause cannot be over-estimated at a time when admission rates to hospital for alcohol-related problems and the incidence of alcoholic cirrhosis have doubled in the last ten years. Up to 30% of attendances at the accident and emergency department may be alcohol-related. It has been shown that a record of the patient's consumption during the previous seven days is a good guide to mean consumption and preferable to asking the patient to estimate for an 'average' day. Alcohol consumption is conveniently expressed in 'units', a half pint of beer, a glass of wine/sherry or a single spirit being a single unit, approximately equal to 10 g alcohol. In men the risks of liver disease increase above a daily consumption of about 60 g alcohol, and in women the corresponding figure may be as low as 30 g. It may be helpful to talk to relatives separately and to look carefully for other possible alcohol-related problems, such as excessive absence from work, accidents, morning sickness, blackouts and depression.

Drugs

Many drugs have been reported to produce occasional adverse hepatic reactions; the most important ones are listed in Table 8.2. They are conveniently divided into predictable (those that

---

Deaths from cirrhosis, due directly to alcohol, have doubled in the last decade

---

Table 8.2   Some drugs associated with jaundice

Predictable
Paracetamol (overdosage)
Intravenous tetracycline
Cytotoxic drugs
Ferrous sulphate (overdosage)
Carbon tetrachloride
Anabolic steroids

Unpredictable
Methyldopa
Antituberculous drugs
Nitrofurantoin
Phenylbutazone
Halothane
Chlorpromazine
Oral contraceptives

will produce liver damage in anyone exposed to a sufficient amount) and unpredictable (where there is an individual idiosyncratic response that is not dose-related). The latter are more difficult to diagnose. An elderly patient on a cocktail of medications can pose a diagnostic problem. It is helpful to remember that most unpredictable drug reactions causing jaundice occur within six weeks of starting treatment.

Biliary tract

Flatulent dyspepsia is common in the absence of significant disease and is therefore of limited use in diagnosing gallstones as a cause of jaundice. However, biliary colic, either in the past or during an episode of jaundice, is a strong pointer towards an obstructing gallstone in the common bile duct. 'Colic' is a misnomer better replaced by spasm, as the pain is constant and severe, usually arising in the right upper quadrant of the abdomen or epigastrium and radiating round to the back or into the chest. It may cause sweating or vomiting, and may last for several hours and can be confused with myocardial infarction. The pain may arise when a stone temporarily impacts in the cystic duct without leaving the gallbladder, hence a history of biliary colic may precede an attack of jaundice by many years. Biliary colic also occurs when a stone migrates into the common bile duct, in which case accompanying jaundice is usual. As the obstruction is often intermittent, so the jaundice is fluctuating. Finally, obstructive jaundice due to stones, unlike that of progressive malignant jaundice, is frequently complicated by attacks of ascending cholangitis that produce fever and rigors. Indeed the combination of severe pain, fever and fluctuating jaundice is almost pathognomonic of a common bile duct calculus. The diagnosis is made all the more likely if there is a past history of cholecystectomy, as up to 10% of these patients will have a residual stone.

The combination of severe pain, fever and fluctuating jaundice is virtually pathognomonic of a common bile duct calculus

Pancreatic disease

Tumours in the head and body of the pancreas produce obstructive jaundice through compression and invasion of the common bile duct at a variable but late stage in the illness; the preceding history is non-specific. Weight loss is usually prominent, partly through anorexia and malabsorption. The classic description of painless jaundice is often not true as pain,

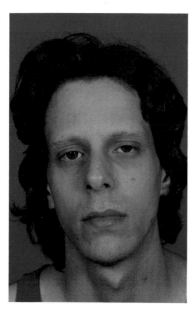

Fig. 8.2   Jaundice.

often nagging in character and felt in the back, features to some degree in 90% of patients. Tumours of the papilla of Vater are much less common but worth detecting because of their earlier presentation and better prognosis. In these patients the jaundice may be fluctuating and there may be accompanying gastrointestinal bleeding. If melaena coexists with steatorrhoea from obstructive jaundice the stool may have an unusual but characteristic silver appearance or 'flash-in-the-pan'.

ABNORMALITIES ON EXAMINATION

General inspection

The presence of jaundice should be confirmed if possible in good daylight. It is most easily detected in the conjunctiva (Fig. 8.2) and buccal mucosa and over the anterior abdominal wall. It is not possible to detect icterus reliably when the serum bilirubin is less than two or three times elevated. Accompanying anaemia suggests haemolysis, particularly if bile is absent from the urine. Anaemia and jaundice may also be seen together in gastrointestinal neoplasia with hepatic metastases and in cirrhosis with gastrointestinal bleeding. A careful search for lymphadenopathy may confirm metastatic carcinoma or a lymphoma. Evidence of recent weight loss may be seen in either cirrhosis or a neoplasm; a rapid deterioration in a known cirrhotic patient suggests a primary liver cancer.

Abdominal examination

After inspection for dilated veins, distension or obvious masses, the liver is palpated beneath the right costal margin. An edge can be felt on full inspiration in normal subjects. Hepatomegaly can be distinguished from downward displacement of the liver, usually by over-inflated lungs, on percussion. The upper border of the liver usually lies in the 5th intercostal space and the vertical span is about 10 cm. The liver almost invariably becomes enlarged in extrahepatic obstruction, is usually enlarged in cirrhosis or hepatic metastases, and is often palpable in hepatitis. The lower border is smooth and tender in hepatitis, but hard and irregular in cirrhosis and metastatic deposits. In the later stages of cirrhosis the liver may become impalpable. There may be tenderness and a friction rub overlying liver metastases, and a bruit suggests a vascular tumour such as primary liver cancer. Clinically it may be difficult or impossible to distinguish cirrhosis from secondary deposits but an enlarged spleen from portal hypertension makes cirrhosis much more likely. Both may produce ascites, presenting with abdominal distension mainly in the flanks and confirmed by the presence of shifting dullness.

Localised tenderness beneath the tip of the right ninth rib suggests acute cholecystitis (Murphy's sign) but is not particularly reliable as it may be mimicked by liver lesions and musculoskeletal conditions. A palpable gallbladder in the presence of jaundice is much more useful and Courvoisier's dictum that this is unlikely to be due to gallstones is rarely proved wrong. The rationale for this is that a gallbladder that has harboured stones is likely to have fibrous thickened walls and be unable to distend sufficiently in the face of extrahepatic obstruction. Thus a palpable gallbladder in the presence of jaundice is usually due to malignant extrahepatic obstruction. Other masses may be palpable, such as pancreatic carcinoma or pseudocyst. A rectal examination not only confirms the pale stool of obstructive jaundice but can also pick up rectal carcinoma presenting with liver deposits.

A palpable gallbladder with jaundice is generally due to malignant extrahepatic obstruction

Stigmata of chronic liver disease

A careful search for extra-abdominal physical signs of cirrhosis may prevent inappropriate investigation or treatment. These are summarised in Fig. 8.3.

Mental state

An alteration in mental state in the patient with jaundice is an ominous sign. Hepatic encephalopathy may occur in viral or drug-induced hepatitis as part of fulminant hepatic failure. Although this occurs in only 1% of patients with viral hepatitis the prognosis is poor. More commonly, encephalopathy complicates cirrhosis, and if related to an obvious precipicating factor, such as sedatives or infection, it may be readily reversible.

Alteration in the mental state of a jaundiced patient is an ominous sign

INVESTIGATIONS

How far a general practitioner will investigate a patient with jaundice depends not only on his personal interest and available facilities, but also on the condition of the patient.

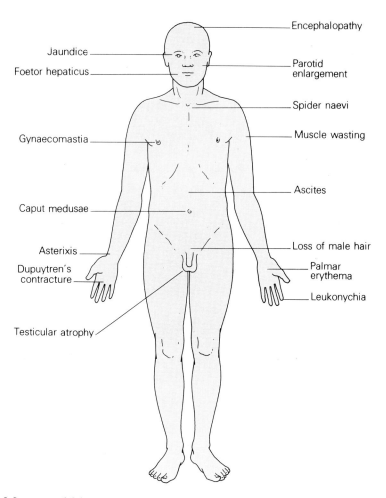

Encephalopathy

Jaundice

Foetor hepaticus

Parotid enlargement

Spider naevi

Gynaecomastia

Muscle wasting

Ascites

Caput medusae

Asterixis

Loss of male hair

Dupuytren's contracture

Palmar erythema

Leukonychia

Testicular atrophy

Fig. 8.3   Physical signs in cirrhosis of the liver.

Most would hope to diagnose and treat at home patients with viral hepatitis if their circumstances allow. Here the relevant investigations are biochemical liver function tests, hepatitis B and Paul Bunnell test. In viral hepatitis the transaminases (ALT, AST) are usually disproportionately raised compared to the serum alkaline phosphatase and are often greater than 1000 IU/litre. HBsAg (the surface antigen component of the type B virus, in the past called 'Australia antigen', Fig. 8.4) should be checked because a small percentage of patients with type B hepatitis may fail to clear the virus and later progress to chronic liver disease. Until recently hepatitis A, the common 'infective hepatitis', was a diagnosis of exclusion, but now it is possible to detect circulating antibody to this virus. To be sure that a positive titre signifies *recent* infection the test should be for IgM antibody to hepatitis A virus. The prothrombin time provides a measure of hepatic function; if it lengthens during an episode of viral hepatitis the patient is severely ill.

Gilbert's syndrome may be simply confirmed by checking that (a) all liver function tests other than bilirubin are normal, (b) serum bilirubin is not grossly raised (less than 90 μmol/l), (c) there is no bile in the urine, (d) there is no evidence of haemolysis on a blood film and (e) the reticulocyte count is not greater than 2%. In occasional difficult cases it may be necessary to refer patients to hospital for provocative tests. Fasting and intravenous nicotinic acid both raise the serum bilirubin in Gilbert's syndrome. Liver histology is normal but liver biopsy should be avoided if possible in this completely benign condition.

Hospital investigations

Further investigation of jaundice usually requires hospital referral to arrange the tests and interpret the results. A flow sheet is suggested in Fig. 8.5. After blood tests the ultrasound examination has a central role, as a skilled radiologist can almost always distinguish 'surgical' obstructive jaundice by the

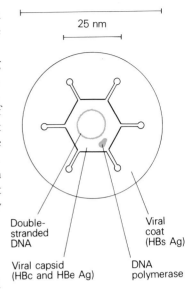

Fig. 8.4 The structure of the hepatitis B virus.

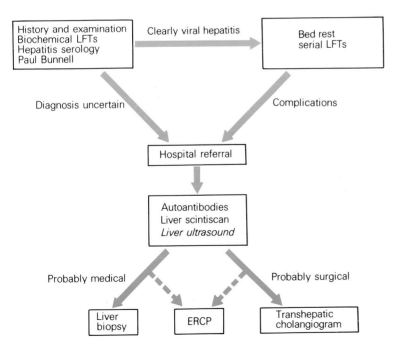

Fig. 8.5 A scheme for the investigation of the jaundiced patient.

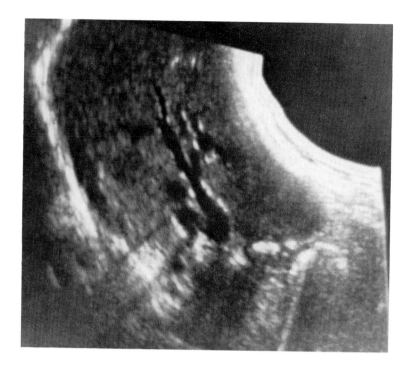

Fig. 8.6   Dilated intrahepatic ducts and a mass at the porta hepatis, shown on ultrasound.

presence of dilated intrahepatic bile ducts (Fig. 8.6). He may even be able to detect the cause, such as gallstones or a pancreatic neoplasm.

If extrahepatic obstruction is demonstrated but the cause is not clear, a cholangiogram will help to plan appropriate surgery (Fig. 8.7). The intravenous cholangiogram is usually unsuccessful in all but the mildest cases of jaundice, and the usual choice is percutaneous cholangiography using a 'skinny' Chiba needle (Fig. 8.8). A biliary radicle is punctured directly under X-ray screening, and the success rate is greater than 90% when the biliary system is dilated.

Retrograde cholangiography through a fibreoptic endoscope positioned close to the papilla of Vater in the duodenum has a comparable success but is more difficult (Fig. 8.9). It is therefore often reserved for cases where percutaneous cholangiography has failed or where the biliary tree is not dilated on ultrasound examination. An exception to this is where the jaundice is suspected to be the result of common bile duct stones, because it is often technically feasible to remove the calculi after an endoscopic sphincterotomy (Fig. 8.10). At the moment most gastroenterologists are reserving this treatment for elderly patients in whom operation is considered

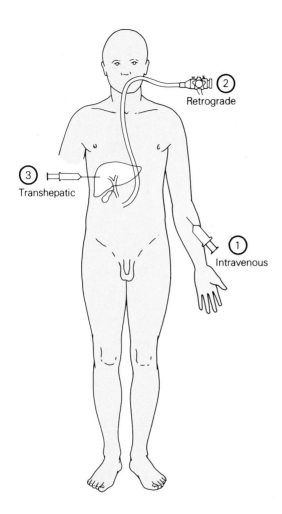

2 Retrograde

3 Transhepatic

1 Intravenous

Fig. 8.7 Approaches to the visualisation of the biliary tree.

unwise, but it might become more widely used in the future. Retrograde cholangiography also has the advantage of directly visualising the papilla and hence diagnosing treatable tumours at that site. The retrograde cholangiogram may also show a pancreatic cancer as the cause of jaundice, although this is likely to be inoperable.

In non-surgical causes of jaundice a radio-isotope scan using ^{99}Tc sulphur colloid is useful in showing filling defects greater than 2 cm in diameter, such as metastases, cysts and abscesses (Fig. 8.11). Also, characteristic patterns of uptake may be seen in widespread hepatocellular disease, such as cirrhosis. Percutaneous liver biopsy is desirable to confirm the diagnosis if there is no impairment of blood coagulation.

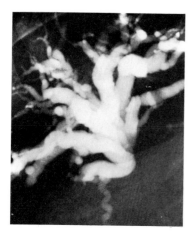

Fig. 8.8 Biliary obstruction due to carcinoma of the bile duct, shown on a percutaneous cholangiogram.

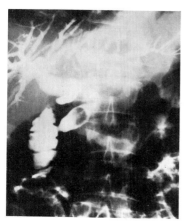

Fig. 8.9 Stones in the common bile duct revealed by endoscopic retrograde cholangiopancreatography (ERCP).

It should be emphasised that there is no place for a speculative laparotomy to establish a diagnosis in the jaundiced patient. Patients with medical jaundice such as viral hepatitis or cirrhosis withstand anaesthesia and surgery badly, and an inappropriate operation has a high mortality. It is almost always possible to define the cause of jaundice accurately, using the above investigations, and to reserve surgery for definitive treatment.

MANAGEMENT

Gilbert's syndrome

It is questionable whether there are any symptoms directly attributable to Gilbert's syndrome. Lassitude and non-specific abdominal symptoms are common, but probably no more so than in the general population. A few patients may get severe unexplained abdominal pain. The serum bilirubin can be lowered by inducing hepatic glucuronyl transferase with phenobarbitone, but this is unlikely to improve well-being. Strong reassurance remains the treatment of choice.

Viral hepatitis

The vast majority of patients recover uneventfully and no specific therapy is indicated. It is important to ensure that every patient's liver function tests return completely to normal; abnormal liver function tests six months after starting an episode of jaundice usually justify a liver biopsy.

Patients with type A hepatitis cease to be infectious soon after becoming jaundiced. Advice about general hygiene and handling excreta should suffice. Those in close contact with the patient during the pre-icteric infectious period can be offered an injection of gammaglobulin (available through the Public Health Laboratory Service). In type B hepatitis patients may carry HBsAg for six to 12 weeks, but are probably infectious only in the first few weeks of the clinical illness, when 'e' antigen can be detected. The position about the family and sexual contacts is not clear, but 'needle-stick' victims should certainly be given hyperimmune globulin. A vaccine for active immunisation against hepatitis B has become available recently and is likely to be offered to high-risk groups such as hospital personnel and the sexual contacts of 'e' antigen-positive patients.

Drug jaundice and unexplained intrahepatic cholestasis

No specific treatment is indicated but it is crucial to withdraw any suspect drug at the first opportunity. To continue taking the drug can be fatal. No other treatment is indicated, and patience is necessary as the jaundice may take several months to clear.

Chronic hepatitis and cirrhosis

Patients who present with jaundice and are found to have autoimmune 'lupoid' chronic active hepatitis respond well to prednisolone 20 mg daily or predisolone 10 mg plus azathioprine 50 mg daily. Drug treatment for hepatitis B chronic active hepatitis is controversial. The rare patients with Wilson's disease respond to the copper chelating agent penicillamine, and removal of iron by venesection remains the mainstay of the treatment for haemochromatosis.

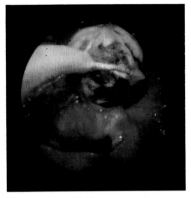

Fig. 8.10 Endoscopic sphincterotomy – cutting the sphincter of Oddi to release gallstones.

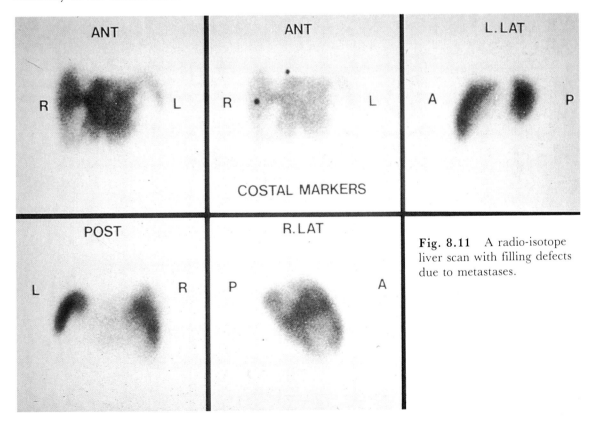

Fig. 8.11 A radio-isotope liver scan with filling defects due to metastases.

The general practitioner is much more likely to be involved in the management of patients with alcoholic liver disease. There is now no doubt that the prognosis is greatly improved by stopping alcohol, and this is central to the patient's management. No 'safe' amount of this liver toxin has been defined and it is safer and simpler to ban alcohol completely. The situation is different in patients with non-alcoholic liver disease, and it seems reasonable to allow them a modest intake. Vitamin supplements, especially B vitamins, are important in alcoholic cirrhosis where diet may be poor. Sedation should be avoided, and indeed all drug treatment should be kept to a minimum because of uncertainty about drug metabolism in cirrhosis.

Diuretics may be needed for ascites, and here spironolactone is the drug of choice in a dose of 25-800 mg daily. There is great individual variation and so treatment should be started with a low dose which can be increased gradually. The peritoneum is capable of reabsorbing a maximum of about 600 ml of ascites daily, and so a weight loss of greater than 0.5 kg per day suggests that diuresis is excessive. The treatment of ascites can often be more dangerous than the ascites itself (see Chapter 10).

Some patients in the United Kingdom with primary biliary cirrhosis are receiving penicillamine. This treatment has not been fully evaluated yet and is best reserved for use under controlled conditions.

Surgical jaundice

Detailed consideration of the surgical approaches to obstructive jaundice is beyond the scope of this chapter. The potential value of endoscopic gallstone removal in the elderly to avoid operation has been mentioned. Many surgeons are not attempting 'curative' surgery in carcinoma of the pancreas, even in apparently operable patients, as the survival rate seems to be no better than that following palliative procedures.

FURTHER READING

Bateson MC (1982) Dissolving gallstones. Br Med J 284: 1-3.

Berk PD, Javitt NB (1978) Hyperbilirubinaemia and cholestasis. Am J Med 64:311-326.

Bouchier IAD (1983) Gallstone dissolving agents. Br Med J 286: 778-780.

Chin J (1982) The use of hepatitis B virus vaccine. N Engl J Med 307: 678-679.

Dienstag JL (1980) Non A non B hepatitis. Adv Intern Med 26: 115-129.

Editorial (1981) Why treat cirrhosis? Br Med J 283: 338.

Editorial (1981) Primary biliary cirrhosis. Br Med J 283: 514.

Leading Article (1977) Are liver function tests outmoded? Br Med J 2: 75-76.

Leading Article (1979) Diagnosis of cholestasis. Br Med J 1: 232.

Machell R, Hunter J (1978) Drugs and the liver. Hospital Update Nov: 688-697.

Scharschmidt BF, Goldberg HI, Schmid R (1983) Approach to the patient with cholestatic jaundice. N Engl J Med 308: 1515-1519.

Welch CE, Malt RA (1983) Abdominal surgery, part 2. N Engl J Med 308: 685-695.

Zuckerman AJ (1979) Specific serological diagnosis of vital hepatitis. Br Med J 2: 84-86.

PAUL M. SMITH

9

Doctor, I've got a big liver

Although it is unusual for a patient to self-diagnose that he has an enlarged liver, physical examination of virtually any patient may reveal the enlarged organ. A big liver is always a cause for concern.

DIFFERENTIAL DIAGNOSIS

The big liver may be due to *malignancy:* liver metastases are a terminal event in many malignant disorders. Primary liver carcinoma is not common in Britain, but it can arise as a complication of cirrhosis or chronic hepatitis B infection. *Cirrhosis* is the second most important cause of hepatomegaly. Over half the cirrhotics in England and Wales are alcoholic in origin, a proportion that is rising as the consumption of beer, wines and spirits increases. Other types of cirrhosis may also cause hepatomegaly.

Big livers can also occur in patients with chronic *right-sided heart failure.* The liver may pulsate, but it will shrink on treatment with diuretics. In contrast, *hepatitis* usually causes only slight liver enlargement, with resolution as the jaundice fades unless chronic disease develops.

Blood dyscrasias, such as myeloid leukaemia, may be associated with hepatomegaly; the spleen will also be enlarged. Congenital haemolytic anaemias and polycythaemia rubra vera can also cause hepatosplenomegaly. In rural parts of Britain *hydatid cysts* can produce hepatic enlargement. Amoebic or pyogenic *abscesses* must be considered if a fever and rigors are present in a patient with a large tender liver and severe constitutional upset. With the growth of air travel, *tropical causes* of hepatomegaly may be seen in temperate climates. Although hydatid disease and amoebic liver abscesses are common in the tropics, schistosomiasis and infection with liver flukes must also be considered.

Table 9.1 Causes of a big liver

Malignancy
Cirrhosis
Right-sided heart failure
Blood dyscrasias
Hydatid cyst
Pyogenic liver abscess
Tropical diseases

It is important to realise that the finding of a liver edge below the costal margin does not necessarily indicate liver disease, but may accompany emphysema and downward displacement of the diaphragm. A palpable Riedel's lobe in the right flank, a normal anatomical variant, can also cause diagnostic confusion. The healthy infant has a palpable liver, which disappears beneath the rib cage as the child grows to school age.

CLUES FROM THE HISTORY

If the patient is losing weight, neoplastic hepatic enlargement must be suspected. Anorexia is characteristic of carcinoma of the stomach, but it can develop with any form of carcinomatosis. A history of smoking may suggest a lung primary.

The alcoholic with a big liver is usually reluctant to divulge his true liquor consumption, and the admitted quantity must often be multiplied by a factor of two or three. A more accurate figure may often be obtained from a relative. Clues to heavy drinking come from early-morning dry heaves and shaking hands. A dietary history will show that breakfast is rarely eaten, that lunch consists of a snack, and that only the evening meal is adequate. A social history may include loss of a driving licence or many days, especially Mondays, missed from work.

The alcoholic is usually reluctant to disclose his true liquor consumption

If cirrhosis has already developed, then other clues should be sought from the history. Ankle swelling and ascites will be readily noticed by the patient. On the other hand, he will probably be unaware of loss of body hair, spider naevi, gynaecomastia or liver palms. The jaundice of cirrhosis is usually mild, but may be accompanied by dark urine. Itching and pale stools occur late in alcoholic cirrhosis.

A history of gastrointestinal bleeding should be sought. If cirrhosis is present, then bleeding varices may be responsible, although peptic ulceration is also common in cirrhosis. Has the patient become drowsy after a bleed? This may indicate hepatic encephalopathy. Finally, a story of rapid deterioration in a cirrhotic, often with recent hepatic enlargement, suggests the development of a primary liver cancer. A story of breathlessness, angina, palpitations, oedema or paroxysmal nocturnal dyspnoea in a patient with hepatomegaly will point towards cardiac failure.

A short history of cholestasis is suggestive of hepatitis, which may be related to drugs, virus infection or alcohol, or of carcinoma of the head of the pancreas; jaundice appears only late with secondary deposits in the liver (see Chapter 8).

If hepatitis is suspected, seek a contact history. This may not always be forthcoming, as the incubation period for hepatitis B is long (50-60 days), and the disease is frequently sexually acquired. Drug addicts and homosexuals are particularly at risk; neither group may admit to their proclivities on initial questioning. All forms of hepatitis are commoner in poor countries; a history of recent travel, especially to Africa or Asia, should be looked for. Lastly, some drugs can cause a hepatitic reaction, so carefully check the patient's drug history.

Hepatic abscesses are rare but treatable, and clues from the history must, therefore, not be overlooked. Amoebic abscesses follow infection with *Entamoeba histolytica*, which may have occurred many years earlier while in the tropics. Pyogenic abscesses can complicate gallstones. Is there a history of cholecystitis? Rigors may indicate bacteraemia and abscess. Hydatid cysts are acquired from a dog. Many sufferers do not keep one themselves, infection having taken place many years earlier in childhood from a neighbour's pet. While hydatid disease is common in sheep-farming country, it can be contracted in urban areas too.

Finally, the patient's family history may occasionally provide a clue. While haemochromatosis is a rare cause of cirrhosis with an important genetic component, the commoner autoimmune cirrhosis may be hinted at by a positive family history. Rheumatoid arthritis, thyroid disease, pernicious anaemia and vitiligo are frequent in close relatives, and should be specifically asked for.

ABNORMALITIES ON EXAMINATION

Careful examination of the liver is essential. Record the amount of hepatic enlargement below the costal margin, as this may vary with progression of the disease. Percussion of the chest will exclude downward displacement of the diaphragm, as in emphysema. Metastases appear as knobbles on the liver surface, which is usually smooth but firm in cirrhosis. A pulsating liver occurs in cardiac failure, especially tricuspid incompetence. Tenderness under the right costal margin may be found in hepatitis, and sometimes with a rapidly enlarging hepatoma. Liver tumours occasionally have an audible bruit, or rub on respiration, heard using a stethoscope held over the enlarged liver.

Having ascertained that the liver is enlarged, look for other physical signs that may give a clue to the aetiology. The patient with alcoholic cirrhosis may have the typical cutaneous stigmata: spider naevi (Fig. 9.1), liver palms (Fig. 9.2), loss of body hair, leuconychia (Fig. 9.3), gynaecomastia (Fig. 9.4), mild jaundice and Dupuytren's contractures (Fig. 9.5). Bruising may follow trauma or clotting factor deficiency. Xanthelasma around the eyes or xanthomata on the elbows or skin suggest chronic biliary obstruction and cholesterol retention. Ascites (Fig. 9.4) and ankle oedema accompany decompensated cirrhosis. Alcohol on the breath is an obvious and important clue.

If the patient has cirrhosis, then the signs of encephalopathy should be carefully looked for. The typical coarse hepatic flap is elicited if the arms are held outstretched with the wrists dorsiflexed, and hepatic fetor should not be missed. Disorientation may be present, or the patient may be unable to copy a figure such as a star (constructional apraxia).

Splenic enlargement can occur with blood dyscrasias as well as portal hypertension. Dilated abdominal veins may appear in the latter condition, but a true caput medusa is rarely encountered outside the examination hall!

Having ascertained that the liver is enlarged, look for other signs to give a clue to the aetiology

Fig. 9.1   Spider naevi in alcoholic cirrhosis.

Fig. 9.2   Liver palms in alcoholic cirrhosis.

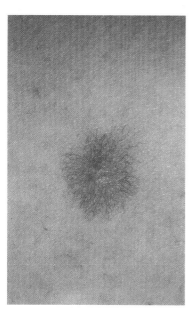

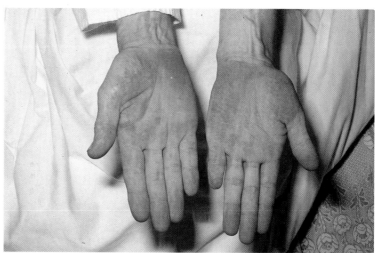

Hepatic enlargement due to secondary carcinoma (Fig. 9.6) is not associated with cutaneous signs of liver disease, but malignant ascites can follow. Sometimes enlarged nodes in the cervical region or axillae may help in reaching a diagnosis. There is often marked weight loss and muscle wasting.

Lastly, do not forget to examine the patient's urine. Bilirubinuria will be present in hepatitis, obstructive jaundice and advanced liver disease. A rectal examination may yield pale stoools, and sometimes a primary rectal carcinoma that has presented with liver secondaries.

INVESTIGATIONS

Liver function tests and a full blood count should be the initial investigations. If anaemia is due to bleeding, hypochromia and a low MCV will be found. If splenic enlargement has resulted in hypersplenism, then the platelet, red cell and white cell counts may all be reduced. A macrocytosis with a normal haemoglobin concentration should arouse suspicions of alcoholism.

Further evidence of alcoholism may be shown by the liver function tests. An elevated gamma glutamyl transpeptidase (GGT), due to enzyme induction by alcohol, may be present (Fig. 9.7). Sometimes the alkaline phosphatase and bilirubin

Fig. 9.3 Leukonychia in cirrhosis.

Fig. 9.4 Ascites and gynaecomastia in liver cirrhosis.

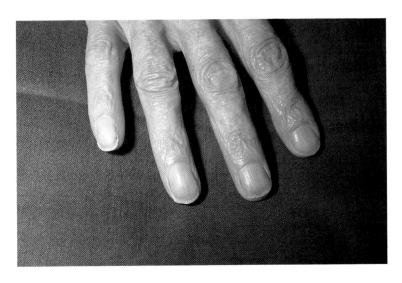

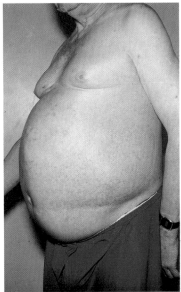

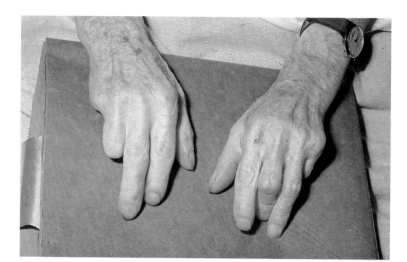

Fig. 9.5 Dupuytren's contractures in alcoholic cirrhosis.

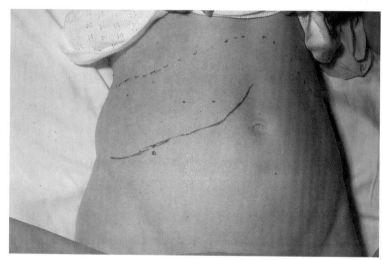

Fig. 9.6 Hepatomegaly and jaundice in a patient with pancreatic carcinoma and metastases.

concentration will also be slightly elevated. Hepatic malignancy is associated with a rise in the alkaline phosphatase and GGT values (Fig. 9.8). Hepatitis, in contrast, is characterised by a very high transaminase concentration, with lesser rises of alkaline phosphatase and bilirubin. Mild cirrhosis may produce little disturbance of the liver function tests, but as the disease progresses the serum albumin may fall with reversal of the albumin/globulin ratio and there may be a slight or moderate increase of bilirubin, alkaline phosphatase, GGT and transaminase concentrations. Hepatic abscesses produce changes similar to those seen with secondary deposits, with high alkaline phosphatase and GGT concentrations.

Presentation	Liver function tests		Diagnosis
A 50-year old man with a long history of alcoholism is seen with ascites	Serum bilirubin	30 µmol/litre	Alcoholic cirrhosis
	Aspartate transaminase	60 IU/litre	
	Alkaline phosphatase	180 IU/litre	
	α-glutamyl trans-peptidase	650 IU/litre	
	Serum albumin	25 g/litre	
	Serum globulin	40 g/litre	

Fig. 9.7   Liver function tests in alcoholic cirrhosis.

Presentation	Liver function tests		Diagnosis
A 55-year old man complains of anorexia and weight loss; his liver is greatly enlarged and is hard	Serum bilirubin	17 µmol/litre	Hepatic metastases
	Aspartate transaminase	30 IU/litre	
	Alkaline phosphatase	520 IU/litre	
	α-glutamyl trans-peptidase	350 IU/litre	
	Serum albumin	35 g/litre	
	Serum globulin	30 g/litre	

Fig. 9.8   Liver function tests in hepatic malignancy.

It is wise to look for hepatitis B surface antigen (formerly known as the Australia antigen) if any primary liver disease is suspected, especially if invasive investigations are contemplated. A chest X-ray will show if the diaphragm is displaced upwards by an enlarged liver; an abdominal X-ray can reveal splenomegaly, radio-opaque gallstones and occasionally calcified hepatic cysts. Isotope and ultrasound scans of the liver may be invaluable. They can detect tumours, abscesses or cysts over 2 cm in diameter (Fig. 9.9), and the enlarged spleen and hepatic abnormalities typical of cirrhosis. Untrasound can also pick up the dilated intrahepatic ducts and gallbladder of extrahepatic biliary obstruction. In a few centres, computerised axial tomography of the upper abdomen can add further information (Fig. 9.10).

Supplementary tests to assist in the diagnosis of space-occupying lesions of the liver include measurement of the serum alpha-fetoprotein, which is elevated in half the patients with primary liver cancer. Hydatid disease can be diagnosed by a positive hydatid complement-fixation test.

If invasive investigations are necessary, then referral to a gastroenterologist is indicated. Liver biopsy can lead to complications, and should be performed only by an

Look for hepatitis B surface antigen if primary liver disease is suspected

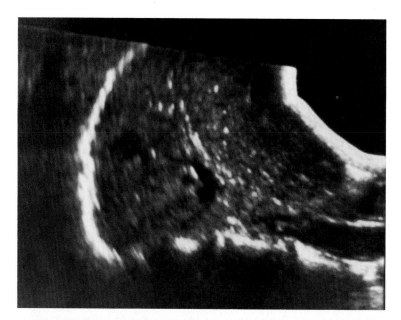

Fig. 9.9 A liver abscess shown on ultrasound.

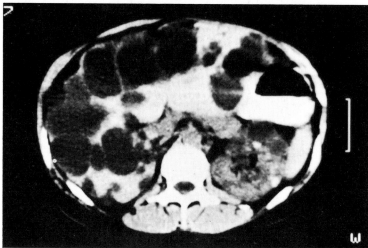

Fig. 9.10 Computerised tomography (CT) – a slice through the epigastrium of a patient with polycystic disease of the liver and kidneys.

experienced physician. Provided that the patient's prothrombin time and platelet count are normal, however, it can provide a definitive histological diagnosis. The accuracy can be further improved by directing the needle with ultrasound towards a solitary tumour.

A barium swallow can demonstrate oesophageal varices in 80% of patients with portal hypertension, and should always be requested if there is a possibility of cirrhosis. Endoscopy is more accurate at detecting varices and provides a route for treatment by sclerotherapy, although this new technique is limited to specialist gastroenterology centres.

Skilled radiological procedures, such as hepatic arteriography, can show the characteristic tumour circulation of malignant hepatic tumours (Fig. 9.11); if the catheter is left in the hepatic artery, it provides a route for infusion of cytotoxic drugs. Splenic venography or superior mesenteric arteriography will outline the portal circulation, and display the collateral circulation of portal hypertension or possibly extrahepatic portal vein obstruction.

Laparoscopy is practised by some gastroenterologists. It allows, under local or general anaethesia, an examination to be made of the the liver (Fig. 9.12), spleen, gallbladder and sometimes pancreas. Target biopsies of small solitary lesions in the liver are possible: it can provide a speedy tissue diagnosis of liver metastases with a minimum of trouble for the patient.

Fig. 9.11 A hepatic arteriogram showing multiple blushes in the liver due to tumours.

Fig. 9.12 Liver metastases observed during laparoscopy under local anaesthesia.

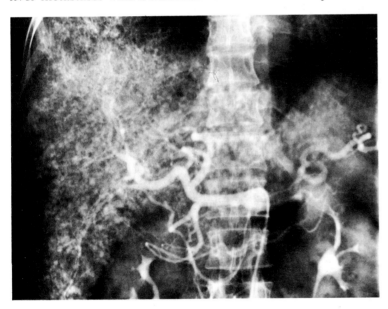

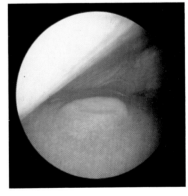

MANAGEMENT

Malignant disease of the liver can be cured only by liver resection or transplantation, which is rarely feasible. Cytotoxic drugs can palliate, but may have side effects. Aggressive treatment, such as hepatic artery ligation or embolisation, should be reserved for those patients with moderate or severe abdominal pain. For the majority, analgesia is the only practical therapy.

For malignant disease of the liver analgesia is generally the only practical therapy

Cirrhosis cannot be reversed but further liver damage can be prevented

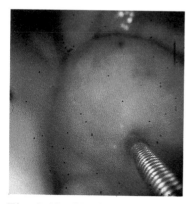

Fig. 9.13 Needle injection of oesophageal varices with sclerosant solution.

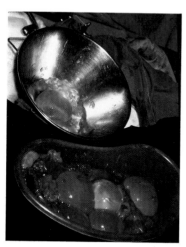

Fig. 9.14 Enucleation of hydatid liver cysts.

Cirrhosis cannot be reversed, but further liver damage can be prevented. The alcoholic may do well if he abstains, but will require careful and sympathetic management to achieve this. Chronic active hepatitis, if hepatitis B antigen negative, will respond well to prednisone. A dose sufficient to suppress disease activity and maintain normal liver function tests will average 5-15 mg/day. In the great majority, treatment must be continued for life. There is some evidence that penicillamine in a dose of 500 mg/day will arrest the progress of primary biliary cirrhosis, but this is not yet widely accepted and further clinical trials are required. Venesection until iron deficiency is produced is effective in haemochromatosis.

The complications of cirrhosis include ascites, encephalopathy, bleeding varices and hepatoma formation. Each is best treated by an experienced physician, usually in hospital, but the general practitioner has an important role to play in follow-up. The management of ascites is difficult, with much scope for doctor-induced disease (see Chapter 10).

Hepatic encephalopathy can be chronic or acute. Acute coma or pre-coma is usually precipitated by a gastrointestinal bleed, which will necessitate urgent hospital admission. A deterioration of hepatic encephalopathy may also be produced by infection, any sedative drug, a high protein intake or hypokalaemia. Purging the bowel to empty any blood, feeding with intravenous 10-20% glucose and oral neomycin or lactulose will be required until recovery occurs. Chronic encephalopathy may be characterised by odd behaviour, euphoria or drowsiness. The basic long-term treatment is to reduce dietary protein intake to 40 g a day, with oral lactulose in a dose sufficient to produce two soft stools each day.

Acute variceal bleeding is a medical emergency. Resuscitation in hospital should be followed by endoscopy to confirm the site of bleeding, and local measures to control the bleeding, such as balloon tamponage. Treatment to prevent later episodes of haemorrhage now includes endoscopic sclerotherapy of the varices (Fig. 9.13), which is replacing the older surgical technique of portacaval shunt (see Chapter 5).

The treatment of hepatic cysts and abscesses will depend on their aetiology. Hydatid abscesses are best dealt with surgically (Fig. 9.14), since effective medical treatment has not yet been established. Amoebic abscesses respond well to metronidazole 800 mg three times a day for 10 days. Pyogenic abscesses can be treated by percutaneous aspiration and antibiotic therapy; if they are secondary to gallstones obstructing the biliary tree, biliary surgery will be required as well.

FURTHER READING

Clark ML (1982) Portal hypertension. J R Soc Med 75: 761.

Conn HO (1977) Diuresis of ascites: fraught with or free from hazard. Gastroenterology 73: 619.

Pande NV, Resnick RH, Yee W et al (1978) Cirrhotic portal hypertension: morbidity of continued alcoholism. Gastroenterology 74: 64.

Sherlock S (1981) Diseases of the Liver and Biliary System, 6th ed. Oxford: Blackwell Scientific.

Vicary FR (1977) Ultrasound and gastroenterology. Gut 18: 386.

Doctor, my tummy is getting bigger

10

With the exception of antenatal patients, the specific complaint of progressive enlargement of the abdomen is uncommon in general practice. It is a complaint that should always be taken seriously because, apart from the increase in girth caused by excess abdominal wind, constipation and adipose tissue, it will usually represent serious disease. Simple questioning and examination will usually detect the presence of excess flatus, faeces, fat and, of course, a foetus, whereas detection of intra-abdominal fluid or ascites can be difficult and yet it is always an important finding.

Detection of ascites is always an important finding

DIFFERENTIAL DIAGNOSIS

The causes of ascites are listed in Table 10.1. Liver disease is the commonest, while other relatively common causes include abdominal malignancies, cardiac failure, intra-abdominal tuberculosis, nephrotic syndrome and, in the world as a whole, malnutrition. When constrictive pericarditis was a more common problem ascites was a frequent sequel.

Ascites may occur as a complication of acute pancreatitis and with chronic pancreatic disease, especially in association with pseudocyst. This is usually referred to as pancreatic ascites and it occurs predominantly in alcoholics.

Rare causes include hypothyroidism and systemic lupus erythematosus. A large ovarian cyst can be mistaken for for ascites, even after an apparently diagnostic 'paracentesis', taking fluid from the cyst.

The presence of ascites in patients with cirrhosis indicates a poor prognosis, with around 25% not surviving more than one year. Ascites may arise spontaneously in these patients or be precipitated by an event that causes more impairment of liver

Ascites in patients with cirrhosis indicates a poor prognosis: 25% survive less than one year

Table 10.1 Causes of ascites

Transudates	Exudates	Miscellaneous
Hypoalbuminaemia:	Inflammatory diseases:	Vasculitis:
nephrotic syndrome	tuberculosis	systemic lupus
malnutrition	pancreatitis	erythematosus
High central venous	Malignant diseases:	Henoch-Schonlein
pressure:	metastases (liver or	purpura
congestive cardiac failure	peritoneum)	Meig's syndrome
tricuspid incompetence	lymphomas	Hypothyroidism
constrictive pericarditis	leukaemias	Whipple's disease
Hepatic venous obstruction:	hepatic:	Pseudomyxoma peritonei
inferior vena cava	hepatocellular	
obstruction	carcinoma	
hepatic vein obstruction	cholangiocarcinoma	
(Budd-Chiari syndrome)		
Chronic liver disease with	Chylous	
portal hypertension	Mediastinal tumours	
Hepatic infiltration:	Thoracic duct trauma	
granulomatous disease	Filariasis	
malignant disease		

function, such as acute gastrointestinal haemorrhage, infection or a primary liver carcinoma.

ABNORMALITIES ON EXAMINATION

Abdominal findings

The abdominal findings vary with the amount of ascites. The distension is due not only to fluid but to gas in the bowel which, in the supine position, floats on the fluid. The umbilicus can be everted and the increased intra-abdominal pressure makes hernias protrude, most typically umbilical hernias. Typically, with the patient supine the flanks appear full and are dull to percussion (Fig. 10.1). When the patient assumes a lateral position the upper flank becomes resonant (shifting dullness). A minimum of about 2 litres of ascites can be detected in this way, whereas much less can be detected by percussing the dependent abdomen with the patient kneeling on 'all fours' (Fig. 10.2).

With tense ascites a fluid thrill is characteristic. Under these circumstances abdominal organs are difficult to palpate, but with moderate amounts of ascites it may be possible to ballotte

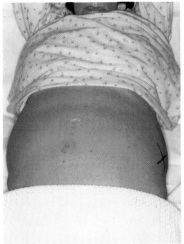

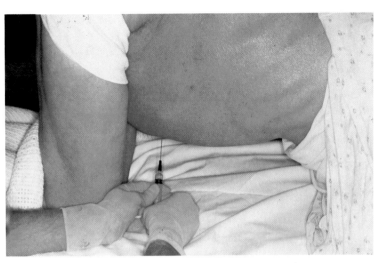

Fig. 10.1   An ascitic abdomen in the supine position showing typical fullness in the flanks.

Fig. 10.2   The patient kneeling on all fours to facilitate detection of a small amount of ascites, which can then be aspirated from the most dependent part of the abdomen.

organs such as the liver and spleen by sharp pressure on the abdominal wall to meet these organs as they move down during inspiration. By this action the liver and spleen are pushed away from the anterior abdominal wall but float back to meet the palpating hand. A doughy feel to the ascitic abdomen is typical of peritoneal tuberculosis. This is the result of loops of bowel becoming adherent to each other and to the anterior abdominal wall. When the ascites are due to malignant infiltration of the peritoneum it is sometimes possible to palpate the peritoneal deposits if the ascites is not tense.

Distended abdominal wall veins which radiate from the umbilicus may indicate portal hypertension (Fig. 10.3). However, inferior vena caval collaterals drain from the groin to the costal margin, or in the flank, and may be due to either an organic obstruction to or a functional block of the inferior vena cava. Carcinoma of the kidney with spread along the renal vein to the inferior vena cava provides an example of organic obstruction, while a functional block can be caused by tense ascites occurring with cirrhosis.

Mild abdominal pain or tenderness, fever or reduced bowel sounds can be a manifestation of bacterial peritonitis. This type of peritonitis arises spontaneously in patients with ascites without warning of, or specific causes for, the infection. This is quite unlike conventional peritonitis (see Chapter 7).

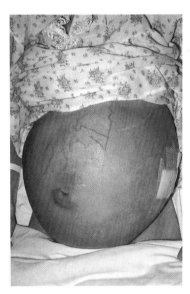

Fig. 10.3   Distended abdominal wall veins in a patient with tense ascites from cirrhosis and portal hypertension.

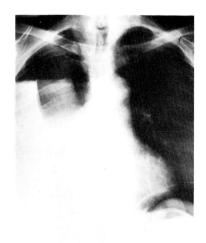

Fig. 10.4 Right-sided pleural effusion in a patient with ascites.

Associated findings

Peripheral oedema is frequently present with ascites but in cirrhosis it is usually less marked than the degree of ascites. Some 10% of patients with ascites have also a pleural effusion, usually right-sided, caused by one or more of a number of mechanisms (Fig. 10.4). These include acquired anatomical defects in the diaphragm and movement of fluid through lymphatics in the diaphragm. When ascites is tense it may impair inflation of the lungs, causing basal pulmonary atelectasis. In constrictive pericarditis, the jugular venous pressure is usually raised. If the ascites is due to cirrhosis all the other stigmata of chronic liver disease may be seen (see Chapter 8).

INVESTIGATIONS

The presence of ascites demands investigation. The single most useful test is a diagnostic tap, when only 10-20 ml of ascitic fluid is aspirated through a 21 gauge needle inserted in the flank, preferably the left (Fig. 10.5). To prevent leakage of ascites through the puncture site after withdrawal of the needle it is worth Z-tracking the needle on its passage through the abdominal wall. This is achieved by drawing the skin over the deep layers of the abdominal wall once the tip of the needle has been inserted into the subcutaneous tissues and before it is advanced into the peritoneal cavity. On removing the needle the skin of the abdominal wall recoils so that the two puncture sites are no longer in direct communication with each other. The aspiration must be performed with scrupulous aseptic technique, usually in hospital.

Macroscopic abnormalities include blood-staining, turbidity and chylous ascites. Uniform blood-stained ascites indicates malignancy, including primary liver carcinoma; turbidity usually implies bacterial infection, including tuberculosis; chylous ascites is caused by lymphatic obstruction and is usually due to lymphoma.

Measuring the protein content of the fluid indicates whether the ascites is an exudate or a transudate. In uncomplicated cirrhosis the ascites is usually a transudate with a protein concentration greater than 25 g/litre but it can be higher, especially during diuretic therapy. The protein concentration is almost always more than 30 g/litre in the exudative ascitic fluid of tuberculous peritonitis and it is frequently this high with

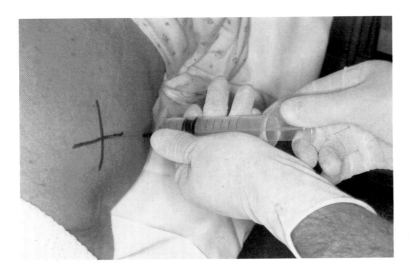

Fig. 10.5   The optimum site for a diagnostic tap of ascitic fluid from the left flank using a 21 gauge needle.

peritoneal malignancy. 'Pancreatic ascites' is also associated with a high protein concentration, but of more diagnostic importance is an extremely high ascitic amylase.

Microscopic examination is also of value. With spontaneous bacterial peritonitis excessive polymorphs are found, while with tuberculous infection an excess of lymphocytes is seen in the ascitic fluid. A search for malignant cells is sensible but is not often productive, unless the sediment of large volumes of centrifuged ascites is examined. Microbiological examination may grow the offending organism in spontaneous bacterial peritonitis, particularly if the ascitic fluid is put into a blood culture bottle (Fig. 10.6), but it is not usually helpful in tuberculous peritonitis. Instead, histological examination of a biopsied peritoneal tubercle will usually show the characteristic caseating granulomata of tuberculosis.

When the presence of ascites is suspected but not proven, even after a failed attempt at diagnostic paracentesis, abdominal ultrasound or computerised axial tomography (CAT) scans of the abdomen can be diagnostic, the fluid showing up clearly against the solid structures like the liver because of its different X-ray and ultrasonic characteristics (Figs 10.7, 10.8).

Having demonstrated the presence of ascites, further investigation is usually required to determine the nature of the associated disease. Usually the primary problem is in the liver (see Chapters 8 and 9).

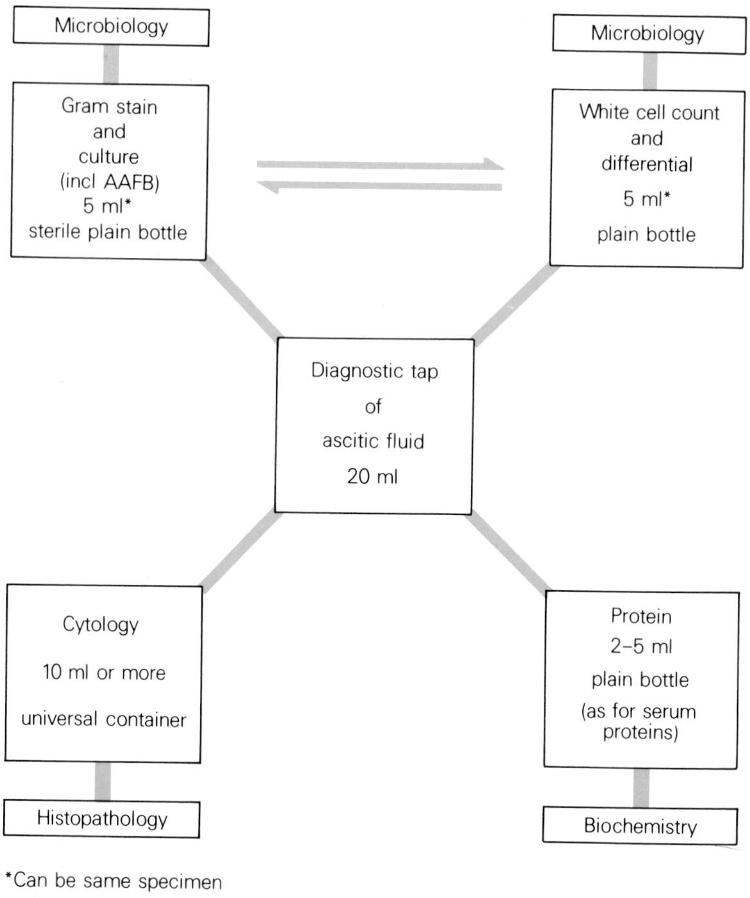

Fig. 10.6 Preparation of a sample of ascitic fluid.

*Can be same specimen

MANAGEMENT

Ascites due to cirrhosis

The main reasons for treating ascites in cirrhosis are cosmetic and to relieve discomfort. Ascites will sometimes resolve spontaneously with improvement in hepatic function when, for example, chronic hepatitis is treated with corticosteroids. Most patients, however, require specific treatment in the form of dietary sodium restriction and diuretics.

DIETARY SODIUM RESTRICTION. A 'no-added-salt diet', together with avoidance of obviously salty foods, reduces the daily sodium intake to 50 mmol. This is usually sufficient restriction but it may be necessary to reduce the daily intake to 20 mmol by avoidance of salt in cooking and the use of sodium-

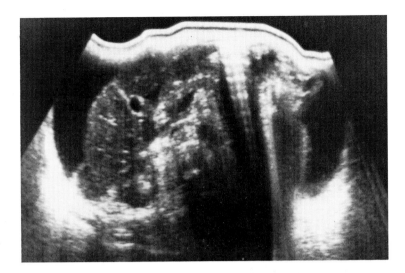

Fig. 10.7 Longitudinal ultrasound scan of the upper abdomen, showing ascites between the liver and the diaphragm and displacing the liver downwards.

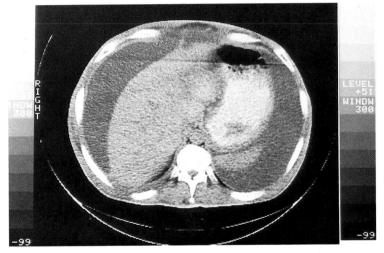

Fig. 10.8 Transverse cut of the abdomen from a CT scan, showing ascites surrounding the liver and other structures.

free foods. It should be remembered that some medications contain sodium or induce sodium retention and their prescription should be avoided if at all possible (Table 10.2).

DIURETICS. Three groups of diuretics can be used: thiazides, loop diuretics and potassium-sparing diuretics. Thiazides include bendrofluazide, chlorothiazide and hydro-chlorothiazide. The loop diuretics are the most powerful and include frusemide and bumetanide. The potassium-sparing diuretics include spironolactone, amiloride and triamterene. The latter group are the first-line diuretics for ascites.

Table 10.2   Drugs with a high sodium content or which induce sodium retention

High sodium content
Antacids:
    Bisodol
    Gaviscon
    Gelusil
Alginates
Antibiotics:
    benzylpenicillin
    ampicillin
    cloxacillin
    cephradine
    cefuroxime
    chloramphenicol
Para-aminosalicylate
Phenytoin
Sodium valproate
Fybogel

Induce sodium retention
Carbenoxolone
Caved-S
Phenylbutazone
Indomethacin
Propionic acid derivatives:
    ibuprofen
    ketoprofen
Corticosteroids
Oestrogens
Diazoxide

Treatment of ascites can be very dangerous

TREATMENT REGIMENS. Patients with mild ascites can be treated with dietary sodium restriction as out-patients or in general practice. With marked ascites the patient should be admitted to hospital. Sodium restriction and bed rest should be tried for three days after admission; if this is not successful diuretics will be necessary.

Careful monitoring of diuretic treatment is essential. Daily measurements of body weight should be made and weight loss should not exceed 0.5 kg/day, unless there is marked peripheral oedema, when a more rapid weight loss of about 1 kg/day is acceptable. Daily weighing is usually more accurate and less cumbersome than fluid input and urine output measurements. Plasma concentrations of sodium, potassium and urea should be checked twice weekly, looking for hyponatraemia, hypokalaemia, hyperkalaemia or a rising urea. A 24-hour urine collection for sodium estimation on admission provides good prognostic information; if less than 10 mmol/day the ascites may be resistant to treatment.

It is really more logical to start diuretic therapy with a potassium-sparing diuretic, because of the importance of aldosterone and enhanced sodium reabsorption in patients with cirrhosis and ascites. Spironolactone has been the most extensively studied and is the most widely used, but it has the disadvantage that it causes gynaecomastia in cirrhotic men. The starting dose should be 100 mg daily. There is usually a delay of several days before the full effect is seen and so the dosage should not be increased more frequently than every third day. The daily dosage can be steadily increased to 300 mg if required. Triamterene and amiloride are also effective in doses of 100-500 mg/day and 10-60 mg/day respectively. Potassium supplements are not required with any of these three diuretics and 'salt substitutes', which are mostly potassium salts, should be avoided.

When a distal or potassium-sparing diuretic is insufficiently effective a more powerful loop diuretic should be added. Frusemide is most commonly used in a starting dose of 40 mg/day increasing slowly to 120 mg/day. Potassium supplements are sometimes necessary despite the simultaneous use of a potassium-sparing diuretic.

Treatment of ascites can be very dangerous: therapy must be stopped if the patient develops hepatic pre-coma (a flap), hyponatraemia, hypokalaemia or a rising plasma urea or is losing more than 0.5 kg/day.

The aim of diuretic treatment is to reduce the amount of

ascites so that it is just clinically detectable. Maintenance therapy is then continued in doses that may be considerably less than those used initially. It is often possible to maintain a patient on a potassium-sparing diuretic alone or to change from a loop diuretic to a thiazide. The patient should be encouraged to weigh himself at home and taught to adjust the doses appropriately. Plasma electrolyte and urea estimations can be measured at intervals of one or two months.

Paracentesis

Paracentesis (draining off all the ascites with a cannula) is an ineffective treatment as the ascites reaccumulate within a few days. It is also wasteful of protein and if large amounts of ascites are drained (more than 8 litres) oliguria, uraemia, hyponatraemia, haemoconcentration and death may follow.

On the other hand, paracentesis can be useful to relieve cardiorespiratory difficulty in patients with massive, tense ascites, especially when this is a complication of congestive cardiac failure, when ascites is associated with pleural effusions or when the patient is in the terminal stages of a malignant illness (Fig. 10.9). The removal of up to 5 litres of ascitic fluid over 60-90 minutes is usually without risk in such patients; it will generally relieve respiratory embarrassment as well as improve cardiac output. This practice can be repeated on alternate days if required, usually removing 2 or 3 litres of ascitic fluid each time. It must not be performed in cirrhotic patients.

Paracentesis is ineffective: ascites reaccumulate within a few days

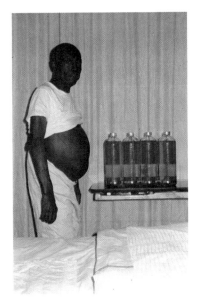

Fig. 10.9 Therapeutic paracentesis (8 litres) in a patient with intractable ascites.

Intractable ascites

Ascites that cannot be controlled by the treatment described above is defined as intractable. Sometimes the definition is spurious because therapy has not been adequate. For example, the patient may knowlingly be taking too much salt; sometimes a drug containing sodium is being given (Table 10.2); or the patient is inadvertently or otherwise taking salt-containing drink or food. Poor compliance with diuretic therapy is another complication, especially when the patient is prescribed a large number of tablets. To improve compliance it may be helpful to distribute the medications more evenly through the day, for example by giving spironolactone at night.

When ascites is genuinely intractable, or responds to large doses of diuretics only at the expense of inducing oliguric renal failure and hepatic encephalopathy, the following treatments might be felt justified:

ALBUMIN. Infusions of salt-poor albumin can produce a diuresis by temporarily increasing a low serum albumin and a low colloid oncotic pressure.

LEVEEN SHUNT. A LeVeen peritoneovenous shunt drains ascites from the peritoneum into the superior vena cava. The shunt comprises a long perforated tube which is placed in the peritoneal cavity, a one-way valve which is placed extraperitoneally and deep to the anterior abdominal muscles, and a silicone rubber tube which passes subcutaneously to the neck where it enters the internal jugular vein and then the superior vena cava (Fig. 10.10). Respiration provides the driving force to carry ascitic fluid into the central vein. Insertion of the LeVeen shunt is not entirely free of complications.

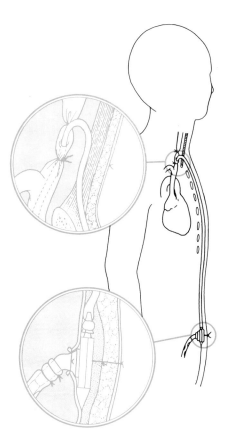

Fig. 10.10 LeVeen peritoneojugular shunt in situ. The two inserts show the valve lying outside the peritoneum and deep to the abdominal muscle and the tip of the tube pushed into the superior vena cava.

Malignant ascites

When ascites is due to infiltration of the peritoneum by malignant deposits or seedlings, the prognosis of the patient is very poor. Treatment is aimed at making the patient comfortable, which means that regular paracentesis will be required. Intraperitoneal instillation of thiotepa has traditionally been used to treat the peritoneal malignancy but this treatment has rarely been helpful. Similarly, diuretics usually have no effect on malignant ascites.

Spontaneous bacterial peritonitis

Spontaneous bacterial peritonitis is characterised by the sudden onset of abdominal pain with rebound tenderness and reduced or absent bowel sounds in a patient with cirrhosis and ascites. However, the signs may be much more subtle, particularly if the infection has precipitated hepatic pre-coma. A fever is usually present and rigors may occur. Hepatic encephalopathy is a common sequel. Sometimes the signs of peritonitis are mild or absent but in the context of a sudden deterioration in a cirrhotic patient's condition, the ascitic fluid should always be examined for infection.

The total and differential white cell count of the ascitic fluid is the quickest approach to diagnosis. The normal maximum concentration of white blood cells in the ascitic fluid is about $350/mm^3$, with polymorphonuclear leucocytes not exceeding 30% of the total count. In patients with spontaneous bacterial peritonitis the total cell count exceeds $350/mm^3$ and the polymorphonuclear leucocytes comprise about 40% of the total count. Bacteriological culture of the ascitic fluid may reveal the infecting organism. The vast majority of cases are caused by a single organism: *Escherichia coli* is responsible for half or more of the cases and the second most frequent organism is *Diplococcus pneumoniae,* which is not an enteric organism. Peripheral blood white cell counts are of no value in differentiating patients with or without spontaneous bacterial peritonitis. Blood culture should always be performed as the organism causing the peritonitis can be found in up to three-quarters of patients.

Patients with characteristic clinical features should be treated with antibiotics immediately, irrespective of the white cell count of the ascites. Likewise, treatment should always be given when bacteria are found in the ascitic fluid even if the patients are asymptomatic. Broad-spectrum antibiotics have to be used until the results of sensitivity tests are available.

Ascitic fluid should always be examined for infection

FURTHER READING

Conn HO (1972) The rational management of ascites. In: Popper H, Schaffner F (eds) Progress in Liver Disease, 4, 269. New York: Grune & Stratton.

Frakes JT (1980) Physiologic considerations in the medical management of ascites. Archs Intern Med 140: 620-626.

Losowsky MS, Scott BB (1973) Ascites and oedema in liver disease. Br Med J 3: 336-338.

Ryan E, Neale G (1980) Tapping ascites. Br Med J 281: 499-500.

Wilkinson SP, Williams R (1979) Ascites, electrolyte disorders and renal failure. In: Wright R, Alberti KGMM, Karran S, Millward-Sadler GH (eds) Liver and Biliary Disease, 1060-1086. London: WB Saunders.

BRIAN GAZZARD

11

Doctor, I've got a big spleen

Normally the spleen is tucked behind the 9th, 10th and 11th ribs on the left and it must enlarge by at least 50% before it becomes palpable. More is probably known about pathological abnormalities of the spleen than about its normal functions. In the foetus and neonate it is an important site of haemopoiesis but not in the adult. The red pulp is the site of degradation of effete red cells and platelets. This is also the site of the removal of inclusions (Howell-Jolly bodies) and nuclei from immature red cells. The white pulp filters lymphocytes from the circulation and probably has important primary immunological functions, although there is no discernable ill health resulting from splenectomy in an adult, except an increased susceptibility to pneumococcal infections.

> The spleen must enlarge by 50% before it becomes palpable

The majority of patients will present in the surgery with features of their primary illness rather than splenomegaly, but a small number will complain of non-specific pain, fullness or a dragging sensation in the left upper quadrant. A few with considerable enlargement will also have vague dyspeptic symptoms from pressure on the stomach. A tiny minority will develop more acute pleuritic-like pain due to splenic infarction which may result from an enlarged spleen outgrowing its blood supply or be a complication of the disease producing the splenomegaly, e.g. bacterial endocarditis.

I am sure everyone remembers the difficulties of palpating an enlarged spleen as a student. Splenomegaly can be one of the most difficult physical signs to detect; the spleen may be soft, the lower end of the ribs may be mistaken for a spleen tip, or the spleen may be so large that it is missed unless palpation is begun in the *right* iliac fossa. Careful studies have now demonstrated that even experienced observers have similar difficulties, and there are wide discrepancies about the degree of splenic enlargement, or even whether it is present or not in individual patients. In difficult patients, palpation is sometimes assisted by turning the patient slightly to the right with the knees slightly flexed, while keeping one's left hand on the costal

> Splenomegaly can be one of the most difficult signs to detect

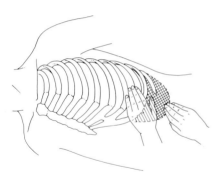

Fig. 11.1 The examination of a patient for splenomegaly.

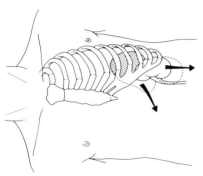

Fig. 11.2 Differentiation between a large left kidney and the spleen.

margin (Fig. 11.1). Sometimes no definite edge can be felt but there is an area of increased resistance in the left upper quadrant which is dull to percussion and contiguous with dullness over the splenic bed. An enlarged left kidney is also difficult to feel and may be even more difficult to distinguish from a big spleen. The direction of enlargement and the ability to feel a space above a big kidney under the costal margin may be helpful (Fig. 11.2). Two time-hallowed physical signs, the splenic notch (usually imaginary) and the band of resonance caused by the colon over a kidney, are, however, not usually of value.

DIFFERENTIAL DIAGNOSIS

About 2% of an unselected group of out-patients had an enlarged spleen, and in a quarter this represented a chance medical finding. Indeed about 2% of normal adults entering further education had splenomegaly, for which no cause was obvious. In some of these cases the splenic enlargement was presumably the result of a previous infection, which was unrecognised at the time. In others a cause became apparent on further follow-up, but a proportion continued in good health for many years with an enlarged spleen.

Although an exhaustive list of the causes of splenomegaly is daunting, the number of diseases commonly encountered in the surgery is small. It is helpful to divide these causes according to the size of the spleen (Table 11.1).

Infection

A whole variety of acute infections produce a soft slight enlargement, which is difficult to feel and usually irrelevant if missed. The two commonly encountered are glandular fever and viral hepatitis. The spleen is notoriously difficult to feel in typhoid fever, but occasionally gives an early clue to the diagnosis of a patient with a high unremitting fever. Similarly, splenomegaly occasionally provides a clue to the earlier diagnosis of bacterial endocarditis, which often presents non-specifically, especially in the elderly.

General practitioners are increasingly exposed to exotic tropical diseases because of foreign visitors, many of whom have enlarged spleens. Malaria is by far the commonest cause, but kala azar, trypanosomiasis and hydatid cysts also occur.

Table 11.1   Causes of splenomegaly

Tip of spleen felt in left upper quadrant
Acute infections: glandular fever
                     hepatitis
                     typhoid
Chronic infections: bacterial endocarditis
                     brucellosis
                     tuberculosis (rarely)
Haematological disorders:
                     megaloblastic and iron-deficiency
                       anaemia
                     polycythaemia
                     myeloma
                     idiopathic thrombocytopenic purpura
Collagen disorders: rheumatoid arthritis
                     lupus erythematosus
Infiltrations: amyloidosis
                     sarcoidosis

Moderately enlarged spleen (to umbilicus)
Portal hypertension
Haemolytic anaemia
Lymphoma and leukaemia

Giant spleen (down to right iliac fossa)
Myelofibrosis
Chronic myeloid leukaemia
Gaucher's disease
Tropical diseases: kala azar
                     malaria
                     trypanosomiasis
                     hydatid

'Tropical splenomegaly' is an esoteric diagnosis reserved for patients with giant spleens and portal hypertension without obvious cause. The majority of such patients, besides a large spleen, also have some degree of fibrosis of the liver producing presinusoidal portal hypertension. The splenomegaly associated with tuberculosis is a reflection of the often widespread dissemination of this infection.

Portal hypertension

The commonest cause of a firm moderately enlarged spleen is portal hypertension, usually caused by cirrhosis.

The commonest cause of a firm, moderately enlarged spleen is portal hypertension

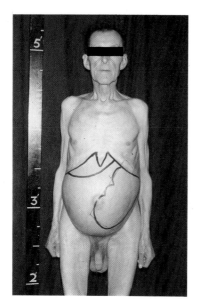

Fig. 11.3 A patient with giant splenomegaly due to myelofibrosis.

Palpation of the spleen is of only secondary importance, but occasionally, particularly in non-cirrhotic conditions, splenomegaly may give the first clue to portal hypertension. Indeed, in one recent study the spleen was always palpable in patients presenting with a haematemesis due to oesophageal varices.

Haematological disorders

The enlargement of the spleen which is seen in haemolytic disorders of any sort is secondary to increased work by the spleen in removing the defective red cells. If the haemolysis is compensated by increased blood production, splenomegaly may be the first clue to the condition.

Splenomegaly is virtually always present in chronic myelofibrosis and is often massive (Fig. 11.3). It is not infrequently the presenting feature of this disease.

Infiltrations

Amyloidosis is not a common condition but involvement of the spleen and liver may be a presenting feature of secondary amyloid where a non-immunoglobulin protein (protein A) is deposited in these organs, in response to a variety of infections. Moderate splenomegaly is present in approximately 10% of patients with sarcoidosis. Gaucher's disease is a common familial disorder in which cerebroside lipids accumulate in the reticuloendothelial system and usually presents as splenomegaly in adulthood.

Neoplastic conditions

The spleen is frequently involved in lymphoreticular and myeloproliferative neoplasms

It is suprising how rarely the spleen is the site of secondary neoplastic deposits. However, the spleen is frequently involved in lymphoreticular and myeloproliferative neoplasms. Perhaps the detection of splenomegaly is of more importance in this group of patients than in any other, as it may represent the first sign of a serious systemic disorder, which responds well to modern chemotherapy. The spleen of patients with chronic myeloid leukaemia may reach a giant size before presentation to the general practitioner with vague non-specific symptoms of ill health.

Trauma

Normally rupture of the spleen follows severe trauma and presents as a surgical emergency. Occasionally the trauma is trivial and even palpation may be sufficient to cause rupture in the enlarged soft spleens of infectious illnesses, particularly glandular fever. Occasionally instead of rupturing completely, the blood may collect beneath the capsule of the spleen and the patient may present in the surgery with an enlarging tender mass in the left upper quadrant. The general practitioner must be aware of the potentially fatal outcome and refer the patient to hospital immediately.

CLUES FROM THE HISTORY AND PHYSICAL EXAMINATION

Infection

Most cases of glandular fever are easily recognised with a characteristic sore throat, malaise, skin rash and fever. A greyish exudate may be seen on the tonsils and petechial haemorrhages of the soft palate are said to be diagnostic. Lymph nodes particularly in the neck are nearly always easily palpable.

Viral hepatitis does not always present with jaundice but may just produce anorexia and fever. An enlarged tender liver is nearly always present.

Brucellosis is usually considered in the context of a pyrexia of unknown origin only in workers in contact with cattle. Occasionally in obscure cases splenomegaly may alert the clinician to the diagnosis.

Patients with typhoid fever are usually obviously ill and in need of urgent hospital referral. The patient is often constipated and frequently the most prominant symptom is headache. This contrasts with the more mild diarrhoeal illnesses of paratyphoid which may also have an enlarged spleen.

Bacterial endocarditis is usually diagnosed because of a combination of fever, a murmur, anaemia, splenomegaly and the presence of red cells in the urine. Increasingly frequently such a classic presentation is absent in the elderly, in immunosuppressed individuals or in those with artificial heart valves. In these patients the diagnosis may be difficult to establish and the presence of splenomegaly is particularly

The classic presentation of subacute bacterial endocarditis is frequently absent in the elderly, in the immunosuppressed and in those with artificial heart valves

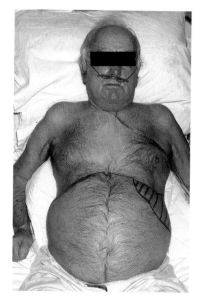

Fig. 11.4 Splenomegaly in a patient with polycythaemia.

important. Rarely bacterial endocarditis is present on a bicuspid aortic valve without a murmur being present and here again the enlarged spleen may alert the general practitioner to the presence of a chronic infection.

The diagnosis of malaria as a cause of an enlarged spleen is usually obvious in patients from an endemic region. Kala azar would not be commonly encountered in general practice but the hyperpigmentation, diurnal fever and giant splenomegaly form a classic triad of symptoms.

Haematological disorders

The symptoms of anaemia usually predominate in the haematological causes of splenomegaly (see Chapter 16), although occasionally splenomegaly is found in the plethoric and lethargic patients with polycythaemia rubra vera (Fig. 11.4). About 10% of patients with idiopathic thrombocytopenic purpura have splenomegaly but again this is overshadowed by widespread petechial haemorrhages into the mucous membranes and skin (Fig. 11.5). A moderately enlarged spleen may be an important indicator of a haemolytic anaemia, although an astute observer should usually be able to detect mild jaundice (Fig. 11.6).

Myelofibrosis not infrequently first presents with giant

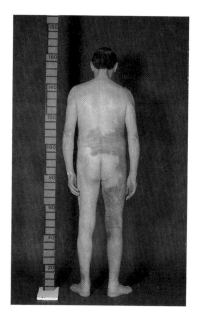

Fig. 11.5 Skin haemorrhages in thrombocytopenia.

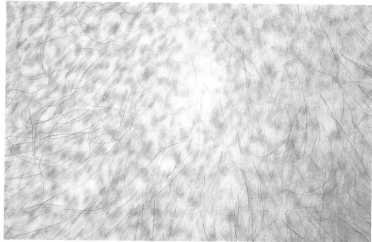

splenomegaly, although patients frequently also have anaemia and have lost weight. Occasionally gout is the first presentation. Splenomegaly is not usually seen in the occasional case of acute myelofibrosis which runs a rapid downhill course.

Collagen disorders

It used to be taught that splenomegaly was a classic feature of disseminated lupus erythematosus, but with more cases being recognised only about 15% have a palpable spleen. Fevers, arthralgias, fatigue and skin rashes are now the common presenting features and the classic butterfly rash, pleural and renal involvement usually occur only in more advanced cases. Felty's syndrome is not really a separate entity but is used to describe patients with the typical erosive arthritis of rheumatoid, who develop splenomegaly and lymphadenopathy with associated haematological manifestations of hypersplenism.

Infiltrations

The manifestations of sarcoidosis are protean and some authors claim that it is supplanting syphilis as the great mimicker. Like the collagen diseases the diagnosis should

Fig. 11.6   Splenomegaly and jaundice in a patient with haemolytic anaemia.

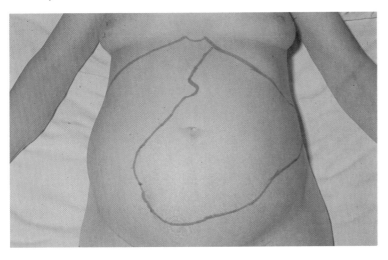

Table 11.2   History and physical examination in important causes of splenomegaly

Recent onset of febrile illness
Glandular fever
Viral hepatitis
(Typhoid)

Well but mildly jaundiced
Haemolytic anaemia
(Pernicious anaemia)

Signs and symptoms of anaemia
Iron deficiency
Myeloblastic anaemia
(Myeloplastic lymphoma)

Symptoms and signs in multiple organs
Disseminated lupus erythematosus
Rheumatoid arthritis (Felty)
Amyloid
Sarcoid

Generally well, non-specific symptoms with or without anaemia or purpura
Lymphoma
Leukaemia
Myeloma
Giant spleen -- myelofibrosis

Perfectly fit, chance finding
Previous infection
Idiopathic: no cause will be found on follow-up
Rarely sarcoid, amyloid, lymphoma
Gaucher's disease

always be considered in patients who present with symptoms referable to more than one organ. It must be exceedingly rare, however, for a patient to present to the GP with splenomegaly as the sole feature of sarcoid. Usually involvement of the spleen with amyloid presents little diagnostic problem as it is secondary to rheumatoid arthritis or a chronic infection, such as bronchiectasis. Kidney involvement with heavy proteinuria and the nephrotic syndrome is a life-threatening complication that must be carefully excluded. Gaucher's disease should be suspected in young fit patients presenting with splenomegaly, particularly if they are Jewish. Additional features may be bone pain, pigmentation and the presence of triangular lipid infiltrations in the corners of the eye growing over the cornea (pingueculae). These are thought to be the remnants of the third eyelid.

Portal hypertension

In most cases of portal hypertension the primary cause will overshadow the symptoms and signs of splenomegaly. A history of excess alcohol consumption, previous jaundice, ascites, haematemesis, together with the stigmata of chronic liver disease, including jaundice, gynaecomastia and spider naevi usually clinch the diagnosis (see Chapter 8). Very occasionally splenomegaly is the only important sign with a non-palpable fibrotic and shrunken liver and no stigmata of chronic liver disease. The other signs of portal hypertension, e.g. dilated umbilical veins (Fig. 11.7) and a venous hum, may help to confirm the cause of splenic enlargement.

Fig. 11.7 Dilated abdominal veins in portal hypertension.

Fig. 11.8 A technetium colloid scan of a patient with an enlarged spleen.

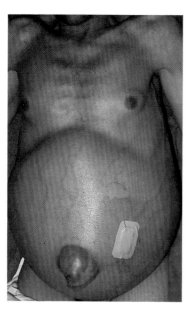

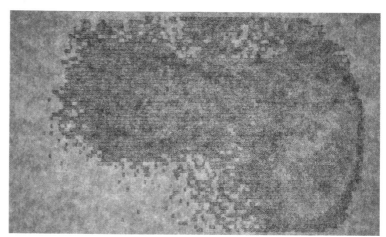

Neoplasia

About 20% of patients with myeloproliferative or lymphoproliferative disorders will have an enlarged spleen at presentation, most commonly with lymphocytic tumours. Unfortunately the presenting features of these important diagnoses are often vague ill-health and it takes an astute practitioner in the middle of a busy surgery to pick up those patients who need physical examination. Bleeding from the gums is always a serious symptom, particularly in children. Systemic manifestations like night sweats, fever and weight loss occur in only a fifth of patients, although most patients with leukaemia will also be anaemic. Many patients will have enlargement of the liver and lymph nodes in addition to splenomegaly.

INVESTIGATIONS

In cases where it is doubtful if the spleen has been felt, a liver-spleen radionuclide scan is a useful investigation. This shows the size of the spleen fairly accurately (Fig. 11.8). It may also show patchy uptake of a radioactive material in the liver, with prominence of the left lobe, suggesting cirrhosis. A plain X-ray of the abdomen may also indicate the size of the spleen (Fig. 11.9).

A liver-spleen radionuclide scan shows the spleen fairly accurately

All patients with splenomegaly require a blood count and film. In a majority of cases this gives a clue to the diagnosis or to the presence of hypersplenism. This is demonstrated by a normochromic normocytic anaemia, a leukopenia (predominantly a reduction in neutrophils) and a moderate thrombocytopenia. This pancytopenia is assumed to be due to 'hypersplenism' if the bone marrow is normal or hyperactive and thus all patients with this blood film should be referred for further investigations. The spleen can be confirmed as the site of the excess destruction of the formed elements of the blood by tagging the patient's red cells with radioactive chromium and scanning over the spleen. Excessive radioactivity over this area confirms that red cells are pooling in the spleen and probably being destroyed. Under certain circumstances splenectomy may then be beneficial.

Further simple investigations depend upon the diagnosis which is suggested after the history has been taken (Fig. 11.10).

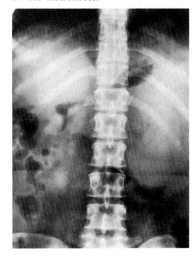

Fig. 11.9   An enlarged spleen shown on a plain X-ray of the abdomen.

Haematological

A marked reduction in platelets probably indicates idiopathic thrombocytopenia and again hospital referral is mandatory.

A haemolytic anaemia is suggested by the presence of fragmented red cells and a high reticulocyte count. Unconjugated hyperbilirubinaemia is nearly always also present. Congenital spherocytosis and eliptocytosis are often suspected on the blood film and an osmotic fragility test will confirm the diagnosis. Hospital referral is usually indicated as some of these patients will benefit from splenectomy.

Myelofibrosis usually presents with moderate anaemia. In contrast to chronic granulocytic leukaemia the Philadelphia chromosome is usually absent and the leucocyte alkaline phosphatase may be normal or raised. Again hospital referral for bone marrow examination is required. Frequently aspiration produces a 'dry tap' and a trephine biopsy is required to show replacement of marrow with fibrosis and the abnormalities of the megakaryocytes which are so typical of this condition.

Infections

In patients with an acute febrile illness, the Paul-Bunnell test detecting a heterophil antibody is usually positive, and atypical mononuclear cells are seen in the blood film of patients suffering from glandular fever (Fig. 11.11). No further

Fig. 11.10 A pathway for simple investigations to be performed on a patient with splenomegaly.

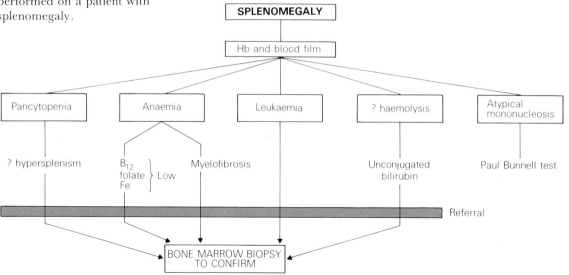

investigations are needed and hospital referral is unnecessary if the course is uncomplicated. Similarly, viral hepatitis is usually easily diagnosed by the presence of urobilinogen in the urine and abnormalities of the liver function tests (raised aspartate and alanine transaminases). Hospital referral is not necessary, but ideally an attempt should be made to determine the virus responsible (see Chapter 8).

All patients with suspected bacterial endocarditis need urgent referral to hospital as early diagnosis has a marked influence on prognosis.

Kala azar can be confirmed by staining parasitised macrophages either from a bone marrow or, if necessary, a splenic puncture.

Portal hypertension

In suspected cases of portal hypertension the liver function tests may be abnormal (although by no means always), and a barium swallow often reveals oseophageal varices. However, hospital referral should usually be considered as a liver biopsy is often indicated to exclude a treatable cause of liver disease and further investigation of the portal system should probably be undertaken. Ultrasound examination will often reveal that the portal tract is patent, thus excluding a portal thrombosis. The portal vein is often also well visualised on the venous phase of a coeliac axis angiogram and only occasionally these days is splenic portography required (Fig. 11.12).

Neoplasia

The majority of leukaemias produce diagnostic abnormalities on the blood film and specialised referral is clearly mandatory. The diagnosis of lymphoma is more difficult to confirm. The blood film is often normal and the bone marrow is involved in only 20% of cases. Lymph node biopsy usually confirms the diagnosis but occasionally the histological type and staging of lymphoma is determined only at splenectomy. A chest X-ray may reveal lymphadenopathy. Early hospital referral is needed for any patient with a suspected lymphoma.

Collagen diseases

Rheumatoid arthritis is confirmed by finding erosions on the radiographs of the joints and usually a positive rheumatoid

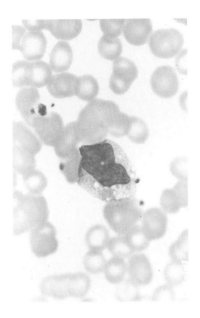

Fig. 11.11 A blood film from a patient with glandular fever, showing an abnormal mononuclear cell.

factor. The antinuclear factor is positive in disseminated lupus, but antibodies to DNA are a more precise diagnostic test.

Infiltrations

As the aetiology of sarcoid is unknown no precise diagnostic test exists. A chest X-ray may reveal hilar lymphadenopathy and occasionally the calcium is raised. Slit-lamp examination of the eye should always be requested. In active disease angiotensin-converting enzyme (ACE) is often raised. In difficult cases biopsy of the conjunctiva or liver may reveal typical granulomas, or a Kveim test may be needed.

Amyloid can be definitely confirmed only histologically and special stains are required. Liver biopsy is more hazardous than in most patients, but may be the only way to obtain the diagnosis. Occasionally rectal biopsy may reveal evidence of amyloid.

Gaucher's disease can be confirmed by finding typical reticular cells with pale cytoplasms consisting of irregular fibrils in a bone marrow biopsy (Fig. 11.13). Patients also have elevated plasma acid phosphatase activity.

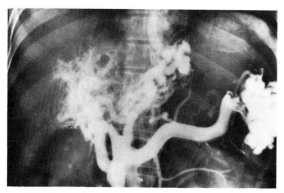
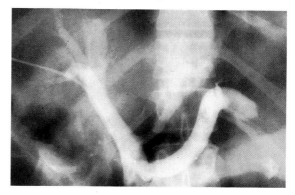
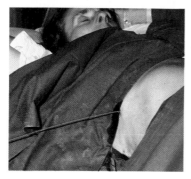

Fig. 11.12 A, A splenoportogram showing an enlarged spleen and oesophageal varices in a patient with portal hypertension. B, The technique of percutaneous transhepatic portography. C, A transhepatic portogram.

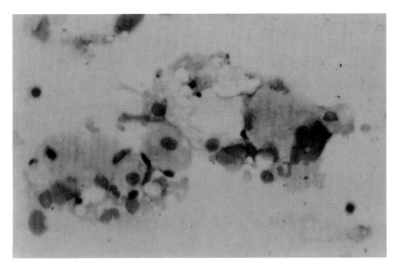

Fig. 11.13   A Gaucher cell in a bone marrow biopsy.

Fig. 11.14   Indications for hospital referral.

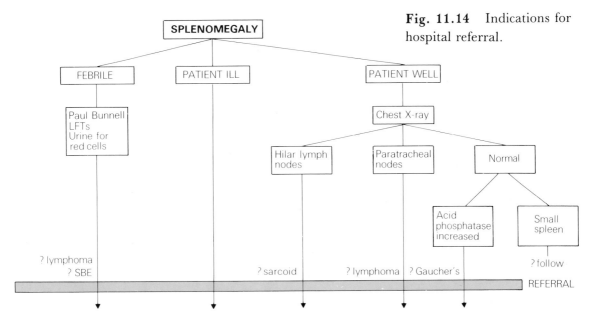

MANAGEMENT

There is not a large place for active treatment of splenomegaly by the general practitioner. Fig. 11.14 shows some of the indications for hospital referral, so that splenectomy may be considered.

There is not a large place for GP treatment of splenomegaly; patients who are referred to hospital require careful follow-up

Table 11.3 Splenectomy indicated if

Usually	*Occasionally*
Symptomatic hypersplenism	Hereditary ellipsocytosis
Chronic idiopathic thrombocytopenia	Giant spleens causing disabling symptoms, e.g. myelosclerosis
Purpura unresponsive to steroids	Acquired haemolytic anaemias when red cells are demonstrably destroyed in the spleen
Hereditary spherocytosis	

Healthy patients with mild splenomegaly and a normal blood film and chest X-ray who are not referred to hospital all require careful follow-up. The splenic enlargement usually disappears quite quickly, but occasionally not for three years. Persistence beyond this time or any enlargement are indications for referral for a specialist opinion.

FURTHER READING

Ferguson A (1982) Hazards of hyposplenism. Br Med J 285: 1375-1376.

McIntyre OR, Ebough FG (1967) Palpable spleens in college freshmen. Ann Intern Med 66: 306.

Schloesser LL (1963) The diagnostic significance of splenomegaly. Am J Med Sci 245: 84.

Welch CE, Malt RA (1983) Abdominal surgery, part 3. N Engl J Med 308: 753-759.

Doctor, I've suddenly got diarrhoea 12

The sudden onset of diarrhoea usually signifies that the patient has developed one of the acute diarrhoeal illnesses described in this chapter. Less commonly, the patient has become aware of one of the chronic forms of diarrhoea discussed in Chapter 13. Although a patient recognise some blood in a diarrhoeal stool (see Chapter 15), bleeding may not be present, or it may be inapparent to the patient, in some of the conditions described in that chapter.

There is sometimes a problem about defining what constitutes diarrhoea. Looseness of stool consistency is the true definition and almost invariably there is an increased frequency of evacuation. The term can range from stools which are just a little loose ('semi-formed') to stools with an unformed watery consistency. The looser the stools, the more severe and uncomfortable is the diarrhoea and the more pronounced its effect on the patient's physiology and symptoms.

	Diarrhoea is a loose stool

It is always useful to have the patient describe the diarrhoea in detail. Are the stools truly watery, or are they just softer than usual? Is there any formed stool at all? Some patients complain of 'diarrhoea' when they simply mean an increase in frequency of normally formed stool, perhaps accompanied by the passage of wind. This may be due to an innocent variation in bowel motility related to a change in diet or to anxiety, or it may herald the onset of diarrhoea in the next few hours or days. Colonic carcinoma may present in this way in the older patient (over the age of about 40 years). Patients with obstructive jaundice whose stools become pale may complain of diarrhoea, but their stools may be soft or loose because of excess fat (due to lack of bile salts as a result of biliary obstruction).

The elderly or neurologically diseased patient can develop overflow 'spurious' diarrhoea in the presence of faecal impaction.

Certain patients are at particular risk when they develop diarrhoea: these patients are more liable to become dangerously dehydrated and to recover more slowly from their diarrhoea. At-risk patients include infants, the very old and the mentally ill; patients with immune deficiency; malnourished patients; and patients who have previously had extensive gut surgery, particularly if they have an ileostomy or colostomy). Many of these patients are residents of hospitals or other institutions, where they are at risk from the rapid spread of food-borne intestinal infections.

DIFFERENTIAL DIAGNOSIS

Table 12.1   Causes of acute diarrhoea

Infections
Drugs and toxins
Intestinal ischaemia
Tumours
Motility disturbances
Inflammatory diseases

Acute diarrhoea can be due to an infection, a non-microbial toxin (e.g. a drug), acute intestinal ischaemia, the development of a tumour or a motility disturbance.

Infections

The principal organisms which cause infection by invasion of the bowel mucosa are the various species of the bacteria *Shigella* and *Campylobacter,* some species of *Salmonella,* and the protozoon *Entamoeba histolytica.* These tend to give rise to bleeding as well as to diarrhoea and are discussed in Chapter 15.

CHOLERA. This infection is normally acquired only in Asia and parts of Africa. *Vibrio cholerae* produce the cholera toxin which blocks the sodium pump (Fig. 12.1) responsible for absorbing

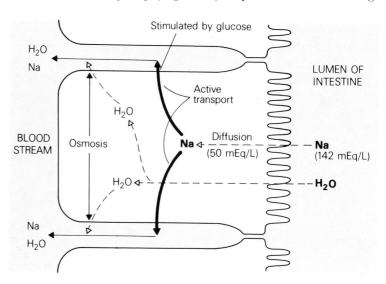

Fig. 12.1   Absorption of sodium through the intestinal epithelium. Note the osmotic absorption of water, i.e. the water follows the sodium through the epithelial membrane.

sodium chloride and water from the small bowel, and this causes a most profuse watery diarrhoea.

GIARDIASIS. *Giardia lamblia* is a protozoon which adheres to the small bowel mucosa (Fig. 12.2), causing malabsorption, often with steatorrhoea, as well as diarrhoea. Although most commonly picked up abroad (visitors to Leningrad are especially prone), it is occasionally acquired in Britain.

YERSINIOSIS. *Yersinia enterocolitica* and *Yersinia pseudotuberculosis* are bacteria which occur from time to time in Britain, usually causing a systemic illness with polyarthritis. They may cause an acute ileitis, mimicking appendicitis or an acute presentation of Crohn's disease; the ileitis may result in acute diarrhoea.

FOOD POISONING. Food poisoning occurring in outbreaks may be due to certain *Salmonella* species or to *Clostridium welchii* Type A, or occasionally to *Vibrio parahaemolyticus;* the latter two organisms produce an enterotoxin with an effect similar to the cholera toxin. *Clostridium difficile* causes pseudomembranous colitis, usually (but not invariably) following treatment with antibiotics. This infection can occur following the use of many antibiotics, especially lincomycin and clindamycin. The organism produces a toxin which damages the colonic epithelium and the diarrhoea is usually accompanied by bleeding.

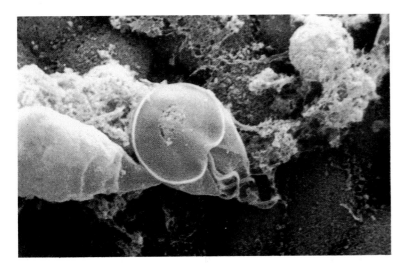

Fig. 12.2 *Giardia lamblia* shown on a scanning electron micrograph.

TRAVELLERS' DIARRHOEA. None of the above infections is the usual cause of the common travellers' diarrhoea, called 'turista' by the Mexicans. This condition is the result of a change in the strains of *Enterobacter coli* inhabiting the gut as a commensal, this change occurring as a result of a varying preponderance of strains in different areas of the world. Some strains product a toxin with effects similar to those of the cholera toxin, giving rise to the well known one- to three-day diarrhoea which travellers so often suffer. These strains are known as toxigenic *E. coli*.

VIRAL GASTROENTERITIS. Some forms of gastroenteritis are viral, due to rotaviruses (Fig. 12.3) which invade the small bowel mucosa and stunt the villi. Children commonly suffer from this form of bowel infection but adults can be affected too. Like the diarrhoea due to *E. coli* toxins, viral gastroenteritis is usually self-limiting, provided the patient does not succumb to dehydration.

Drugs and toxins

Laxative preparations are used to produce purgation. A child may inadvertently take an overdose, especially of chocolate-flavoured laxatives. Some psychiatrically disturbed patients take large amounts of laxatives surrepticiously and patients with anorexia nervosa may also be laxative abusers. The magnesium-containing antacids have a considerable laxative tendency.

Many of the broad-spectrum antibiotics taken orally are liable to cause diarrhoea, and this is only rarely due to classical pseudomembranous colitis. It is presumed that the antibiotics

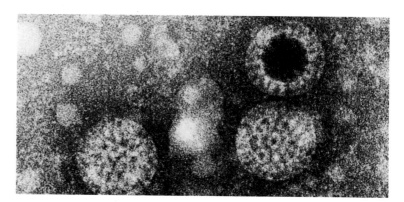

Fig. 12.3 Three rotavirus particles in human faeces shown on an electron micrograph.

cause a change in the intestinal flora. Diarrhoea has been listed as a side effect of many drugs, examples being cimetidine, clofibrate, digoxin and methyldopa, but the diarrhoea is rarely severe.

Intestinal ischaemia

Patients who suffer mesenteric ischaemia or infarction have severe abdominal pain, may be shocked and usually pass blood as well as having diarrhoea. Older patients who suffer an attack of segmental ischaemic colitis present predominantly with rectal bleeding, but they may just report diarrhoea in the early stages or a mild episode.

Tumours

Colonic tumours, especially when mucus-secreting, can present with diarrhoea (Fig. 12.4). The alteration in bowel habit may start insidiously but the patient may become suddenly aware of the diarrhoea, for instance if an intestinal infection is contracted coincidentally. In rare cases of gastric or colonic carcinoma, a gastrocolic fistula may develop, with a sudden onset of diarrhoea due to bacterial colonisation of the small bowel. Similarly, a patient may become suddenly aware of diarrhoea due to one of the rather rare endocrine tumours (carcinoid, VIPoma, gastrinoma).

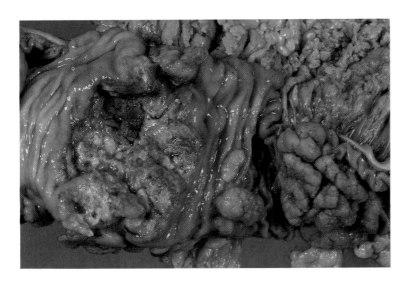

Fig. 12.4 Carcinoma of the colon.

Motility disturbances

The irritable bowel syndrome does not usually present as an acute diarrhoea, except when it follows on a bowel infection or if the patient has become anxious as a result of an acute personal crisis, such as bereavement or a marital or employment problem.

Inflammatory diseases

Ulcerative colitis and Crohn's disease often present as acute diarrhoea. However, bleeding is usually a feature of ulcerative colitis and colonic Crohn's disease, and abdominal pain tends to be present in small intestinal Crohn's disease (see Chapters 13 and 15).

Acute diverticulitis may cause acute diarrhoea with associated fever and tenderness over the infected segment, which is usually in the left iliac fossa.

CLUES FROM THE HISTORY

Patients with acute diarrhoea should always be asked about travel outside the British Isles in the preceding few months. They should also be asked about their diet in the week before the illness, to ascertain whether they have been eating out of their homes or if they have had any unusual foods or undercooked meat or fish. One should enquire of the health of other members of the patient's family and of close colleagues at work. For patients who live or eat in a large institution it may be worth while enquiring of a responsible person at that institution whether there has been any sudden occurrence of gastrointestinal symptoms in others who have been eating there.

Patients should always be asked about the presence of rectal bleeding and the localisation of any abdominal pain. They should be asked about any weight loss preceding the onset of the diarrhoea, in order to uncover a chronic underlying disorder. They should also be asked about any vomiting, a symptom which will usually point to an infection (or occasionally to Crohn's disease). Enquiries should be made regarding previous gastrointestinal diseases and operations.

A drug history should always be taken, together with questions about possible industrial or other exposure to toxic compounds. A patient should be asked if there has been any sudden personal crisis.

One should also enquire if the patient has had any other symptoms, such as joint pains (suggestive of inflammatory bowel disease or *Yersinia* infection) or more generalised complaints like tiredness or shivering.

ABNORMALITIES ON EXAMINATION

Start by looking for signs of dehydration (Fig. 12.5), such as a dry tongue, poor skin turgor, a low blood pressure or a tachycardia disproportionate to the degree of any fever. Always have a general look at the patient to see if there is any anaemia or jaundice. The patient's temperature should be taken; if there is a pyrexia the diagnosis is likely to be one of the infectious causes, although severe inflammatory bowel disease can present with a fever.

An examination of the abdomen should always be performed, palpating for masses due to tumours or Crohn's disease. See if the patient's abdomen is distended, though there are relatively few conditions in the differential diagnosis of diarrhoea which are not capable of giving rise to some distension. Look for scars of previous abdominal operations in case the patient has forgotten to mention them. Listening for bowel sounds will generally be of little help. Listening for abdominal bruits will assist only in the very rare cases of mesenteric ischaemia.

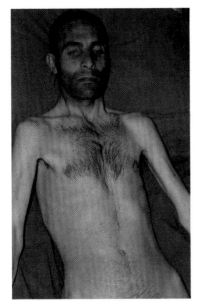

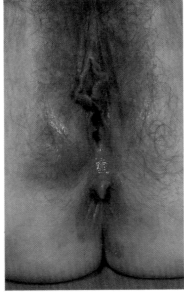

Fig. 12.5 Dehydration.

Fig. 12.6 Perianal skin tags due to Crohn's disease presenting with diarrhoea.

Should a rectal examination be performed? Almost always yes. It is wise to perform a rectal examination to rule out an easily palpable tumour in patients developing diarrhoea over the age of 40 (or even 25, when there is a family history of bowel cancer), and in all patients whose diarrhoea persists for more than a few days. Where there is doubt about the cause of the diarrhoea, even in the first few days of the illness, a rectal examination may reveal the presence of blood which was not observed by the patient. The rectal mucosa may be felt to be granular in ulcerative colitis and sometimes also in other forms of colitis, such as shigellosis. The finding of perianal abscesses, skin tags (Fig. 12.6) or fissures suggests the possibility of Crohn's disease (see Chapter 19). In the elderly, a rectal examination is always necessary to rule out faecal impaction.

INVESTIGATIONS

Stool analysis

Stool samples should be sent to the laboratory as soon as possible

A sample of the stool should be sent to the laboratory for culture as soon as possible. As well as assisting in the diagnosis of an individual patient's diarrhoea, it is also valuable epidemiologically.

The laboratory receiving the specimen needs to be told if the patient has been receiving any antibiotics, if there has been any contact with another person in whom a pathogenic organism has already been found, and if the patient has recently been abroad. In the latter case a fresh stool should be sent to the laboratory to look for parasites; microscopic examination may reveal vegetative forms of *Entamoeba histolytica,* amoebic or other rarer cysts or *Giardia lamblia.* Some laboratories look for pus cells in the stool; these are much more likely to be seen in diseases of colonic inflammation (*Salmonella, Shigella,* acute amoebiasis and ulcerative colitis) than in diarrhoea due to an enterotoxin or a virus.

Testing the stool for occult blood does not help greatly in the assessment of a patient with acute diarrhoea. A young patient whose diarrhoea remits completely will not require further investigations if there are no other symptoms, but it is wise always to consider the possibility of colonic carcinoma in older patients. A positive test for faecal occult blood will indicate the need for further investigation in a borderline patient (for instance, where diarrhoea does not settle after an acute illness).

Faecal fat measurements are used only in the investigation of persistent diarrhoea.

Blood analysis

Severe diarrhoea causes dehydration, raising the serum sodium, urea and creatinine concentrations. Losses of potassium and bicarbonate in diarrhoeal stools cause hypokalaemia and acidosis (with a low serum bicarbonate). The dangers of dehydration are hypotension and renal failure; hypernatraemia can cause confusion and coma; hypokalaemia can induce dangerous cardiac arrhythmias; and acidosis is hazardous in itself.

However, the important decision about whether or not a patient with acute diarrhoea requires admission to hospital must be based on a clinical assessment of the patient. The general practitioner should beware of sending blood to the laboratory to help make this decision. There will almost inevitably be some delay and, if there is sufficient concern to regard these investigations as crucial, this means that referral should be arranged urgently. The blood investigations mentioned are certainly important to the patient's management in hospital, and other blood studies -- particularly the ESR or plasma viscosity, the serum albumin concentration and liver function tests -- may help distinguish cases of diarrhoea which are chronic or superimposed on existing gastrointestinal disease. However, their value in the general practice management of acute diarrhoea is limited.

> The decision on whether or not to admit the patient to hospital must be based on the clinical assessment

Even in the absence of rectal bleeding, a haemoglobin estimation may be useful, revealing anaemia or pointing to serious underlying disease (see Chapter 16). A high white cell count suggests a severe infectious or inflammatory disease.

Sigmoidoscopy

Provided a stool culture and a rectal examination have been performed and there is no bleeding, sigmoidoscopy can be deferred for the first few days of an acute diarrhoeal illness. After this time it is useful to to arrange a sigmoidoscopic examination. However, there is no urgency about this unless the patient's general condition is not improving, in which case there should be referral to hospital, where sigmoidoscopy should always be performed at the time of admission.

> Sigmoidoscopy differentiates rectal and non-rectal causes of diarrhoea

If the practitioner is trained to perform sigmoidoscopy, this simple examination will allow differentiation of rectal and non-rectal causes of the diarrhoea. *Salmonella, Shigella, Campylobacter, Clostridium difficile* (pseudomembranous colitis) and amoebic infections normally involve the rectum (together with the whole large bowel); ulcerative colitis always involves the rectum (with a variable proximal extent); and Crohn's disease may or may not involve the rectum. These diseases cause granularity or ulceration of mucosa of variable type and degree (see Chapter 19). Up to half the carcinomas of the large bowel are in the rectum or sigmoid colon. The rectum is not involved in diseases of the small bowel, which include the enterotoxin-induced infections (*E. coli, Clostridium welchii, Vibrio parahaemolyticus* and *V. cholerae*), rotaviruses, *Yersinia, Giardia lamblia,* and tropical sprue, as well as coeliac disease and dietary intolerance (such as hypolactasia).

The rectum is also unaffected in drug-induced diarrhoeas (other than pseudomembranous colitis), the irritable bowel syndrome or diverticulosis. However, there may be some hyperaemia and mucosal oedema in any patient with severe diarrhoea.

A rectal biopsy should be performed at the same time as the sigmoidoscopy if any abnormality is found or if the appearances are doubtful. This will help to distinguish the various forms of colitis (including the infectious causes). Rectal biopsy should not normally be performed outside a hospital, in case of rare complications.

Doctors performing rectal examination, proctoscopy or sigmoidoscopy should be scrupulous about hygiene, particularly when examining any patient with acute infectious diarrhoea.

Rectal examinations of whatever kind must be conducted with scrupulous attention to hygiene

---

Radiology

A plain abdominal radiograph is not of great help in diagnosing the patient with acute diarrhoea, unless the patient appears so ill as to be a candidate for acute mesenteric ischaemia or for toxic dilatation of the colon; the latter is a relatively rare complication of ulcerative colitis and occasionally of other forms of colitis (including Crohn's and pseudomembraneous colitis). Patients with these conditions are usually toxic and very ill, often with a distended abdomen, and they should always be referred urgently to hospital.

For two clinical reasons a barium enema is not usually carried out until the patient has had diarrhoea for a week or more. An acute infection needs to be excluded before X-ray staff are unnecessarily exposed to the risk of infection and a barium enema is considered by some to be hazardous in acute ulcerative colitis.

The barium enema will not assist in diagnosing an infectious cause of diarrhoea, and it should always be done after a sigmoidoscopy has been performed. It is of the value in diagnosing carcinoma, Crohn's disease or ischaemic colitis and in assessing the severity of ulcerative colitis. It may demonstrate diverticulosis coli in older patients, though this is such a common condition that one should be wary of assuming that diverticulosis is necessarily the cause of the diarrhoea. The barium enema will be normal in the irritable bowel syndrome.

Small bowel barium X-rays should normally be delayed for two or three weeks unless a mass in the right iliac fossa suggests Crohn's disease. Such an examination should always be deferred until infection has been excluded, and it should be performed after a sigmoidoscopy and barium enema unless there are strong clinical or biochemical pointers to small bowel disease.

Small bowel biopsy

Fig. 12.7 A Crosby capsule and an X-ray showing it in position in the upper small intestine.

Biopsies from the most proximal part of the jejunum are taken with a Crosby capsule (Fig. 12.7); they may show abnormalities in coeliac disease, tropical sprue and viral gastroenteritis. The most important of these abnormalities comprise some degree of stunting of the villi. *Giardia lamblia* organisms (when present) can be seen adherent to the villi. Sometimes this is the only way to diagnose giardiasis, as the parasite may not be found in the stool (Fig. 12.8).

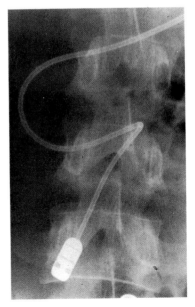

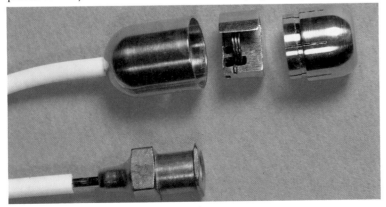

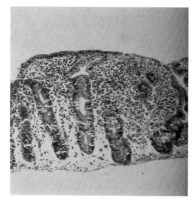

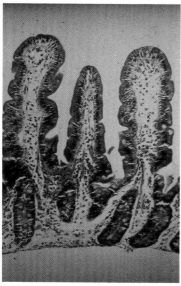

Fig. 12.8   Jejunal biopsy from a patient with giardiasis, before and after treatment with metronidazole. Normal villi return.

These histological diagnoses can also be made on biopsies from the second or third parts of the duodenum, which can be obtained at gastroduodenoscopy with the new, thinner, fibreoptic endoscopes. Small bowel biopsies should not be taken too early in the course of a diarrhoeal illness because viral gastroenteritis is a self-limiting condition which can mimic histologically the milder forms of coeliac disease.

MANAGEMENT

Correction of the effects of diarrhoea

If a patient is severely ill dehydration should be corrected by intravenous fluid replacement in hospital. Milder illnesses can be managed at home, warning the patient and the family about the importance of avoiding dehydration (which will be more likely if the patient is febrile).

Most causes of large-volume acute diarrhoea involve diminished small intestinal absorption of sodium (due to infection, diseases of the small bowel or an enterotoxin). Attention must centre on overcoming this abnormality. Sodium is normally absorbed by the action of a sodium pump (see Fig. 12.1), which is the result of a series of biochemical processes in the small intestinal epithelial cell. This pump requires glucose in order to function normally; it has been discovered that the more glucose there is within the lumen of the small intestine the faster the sodium pump operates. Sucrose (which is less expensive and widely available) has been found to prime the pump as effectively as glucose.

The adult patient should be told to drink large quantities (several litres per day) of water containing plenty of sucrose or glucose, together with some sodium and a little potassium (the latter to replace losses in the stool). Commercial pharmaceutical products are available, such as Dioralyte or Rehydrat sachets (sodium chloride and potassium with sugars, for dilution). These are relatively expensive but are valuable for children in whom the electrolyte and glucose concentrations are more critical than for adults. Most brands of lemonade are effective, though they may be better tolerated if left to go flat. Cola drinks are also used, but these often contain caffeine which has been shown to increase intestinal motility, which is probably counter-productive. Coffee and tea also contain caffeine, but warm, sweetened weak tea can be very palatable and acceptable to an adult patient. All these drinks are virtually salt-free and some kind of salt supplement should also be provided. Weakly salted soups may also be suitable. Fruit juices usually contain potassium salts.

The other components of the diet can be witheld for three or four days to allow diarrhoea to remit (as it will nearly always do if it is viral or due to an enterotoxin). Unabsorbed carbohydrates (those other than glucose, fructose and sucrose) will tend to ferment in the small intestine, the gases of fermentation causing uncomfortable dilatation of the small and large bowel, as well as aggravating the diarrhoea. Many of the transient intestinal infections cause a degree of stunting of the small intestinal villi, resulting in a loss of small intestinal lactase, the enzyme responsible for converting the disaccharide sugar lactose to the monosaccharides glucose and galactose. Thus milk (which contains lactose) should not be fed in large quantities to patients with acute diarrhoea or for a day or two afterwards.

Anti-diarrhoeal drugs

The use of anti-diarrhoeal drugs is widespread but rather controversial. Kaolin and morphine mixture is a traditional remedy, but the newer drugs are all derivatives of morphine: codeine phosphate, diphenoxylate (combined with a small dose of atropine in Lomotil) and loperamide.

Kaolin itself is no longer believed to 'adsorb' bacterial toxins; its value is doubtful but it may help to cause the stools to become a little more bulky as the kaolin molecules hold water. Codeine phosphate, diphenoxylate and loperamide have been shown to be equally effective in equivalent doses (30 mg, 5 mg and 2 mg respectively). Faecal water excretion has been shown to be diminished by their use, though only by a modest factor of about 25%.

Morphine, codeine and diphenoxylate can cause central nervous system depression. Loperamide has no significant central sedative effects and it should have little hazard when taken as an accidental overdose (usually by a child). Such a tragedy is a real danger with diphenoxylate, when less than 10 tablets may be fatal for a child of even six years of age.

When prescribing these drugs the doctor should always consider the cause of the diarrhoea. Anti-diarrhoeals should never be a substitute for fluid and electrolyte replacement. The danger of ignoring dehydration is greatest in children, in whom anti-diarrhoeal drugs are best avoided.

Anti-diarrhoeals must never be a substitute for fluid and electrolyte replacement

Antimicrobial agents

Antimicrobial agents are rarely needed for acute diarrhoeal illnesses!

Samonella typhi infection must be treated only under the direction of a hospital specialist; the effective antibiotics are cotrimoxazole, ampicillin and chloramphenicol. Gastro-enteritis caused by other *Salmonella* species is best treated without antibiotics unless the illness is prolonged or there is evidence of bacteraemia; infection has been shown to be more prolonged in patients treated with antibiotics.

Shigella infections are often resistant to ampicillin and tetracycline, formerly the antibiotics of choice for this group of organisms. Supportive treatment of the diarrhoea is more important in the early stages; antibiotic treatment can wait until the laboratory has isolated the organism and tested for antibiotic sensitivities.

The antibiotic of choice for *Campylobacter* infections is erythromycin, but again the benefit of this treatment is not clear. Erythromycin should be given only to patients with a severe systemic upset, with fever or pain.

Clostridium difficile infection (pseudomembranous colitis) requires specific therapy with vancomycin (see Chapter 15).

Vibrio parahaemolyticus and *Clostridium welchii* food poisoning, together with *toxigenic E. coli* infection, do not require antibiotic therapy, as the patients recover spontaneously with supportive treatment. However, recent American studies showed a more rapid resolution of symptoms when patients with travellers' diarrhoea in Mexico were treated with co-trimoxazole or trimethoprim.

There are, of course, no suitable antimicrobial agents for *viral* gastroenteritis.

Giardia lamblia infection is treated with metronidazole (400 mg 8-hourly for seven days).

Isolation of infected patients

The infectious diarrhoeal diseases are spread by the faecal-oral route. Every patient with acute diarrhoea should observe very strict hygiene until a non-infectious cause is established or the patient has recovered. Patients in institutions with these infections should always be isolated as early as possible. Isolation within a family group may be difficult, but visitors should be discouraged and personal hygiene encouraged.

Prophylactic treatment

The use of prophylactic antimicrobial agents for travellers to prevent infectious diarrhoea is controversial. A number of studies have shown that prophylactic antibiotics will protect travellers from the West when travelling in the more exotic parts of the world. However, the results of such trials may not be reproducible in other populations in other parts of the world. All antibiotics carry a small risk of toxicity, which could well become more apparent if they are prescribed on a large scale to today's millions of international travellers.

Prophylactic treatment with antibiotics should probably be restricted to those few business or diplomatic travellers for whom a short-lived episode of diarrhoea could be a professional disaster. Such patients are probably best treated with prophylactic trimethoprim. Alternatively, they could be provided with a supply of trimethoprim to take at the first signs of any prolonged diarrhoea.

Active immunisation against typhoid fever, paratyphoid A and B and cholera is advisable for persons travelling to the appropriate areas of Africa, Asia and Latin America.

FURTHER READING

Carpenter CCJ (1982) Oral rehydration. Is it as good as parenteral therapy? N Engl J Med 306: 1103-1104.

Gorbach SL (1982) Travelers' diarrhea. N Engl J Med 307: 881-883.

Guerrant RL (1980) Yet another pathogenic mechanism for *Escherichia coli* diarrhoea? N Engl J Med 302: 113-114.

Leading Article (1981) Gastroenteritis in Britain: management at home. Br Med J 283: 1277-1278

Leading Article (1983) Management of acute diarrhoea. Lancet 1: 623-626.

Lissauer T (1982) Paediatric emergencies: diarrhoea and vomiting. Update 5: 1978-1992.

Mandel BK (1981) Intestinal infections in adults and children over the age of two. Med Int 1: 56-61.

Tarlow MJ (1981) Acute infantile gastroenteritis. Med Int 1: 51-55.

Doctor, I often get diarrhoea

There is a wide spectrum of possible diagnoses for the patient who presents with a history of chronic diarrhoea. A functional bowel disorder, the irritable bowel syndrome, will be the commonest final diagnosis; in many patients positive features will allow a quick diagnosis, although in some patients it may have to be a diagnosis of exclusion. Most infective causes of diarrhoea will present as bowel disturbance of sudden onset (see Chapter 12); colonic infections, ulcerative colitis and proctitis are discussed in Chapter 15, although it is as well to remember that the diarrhoea in the inflammatory bowel disorders of the colon may not be overtly bloody.

Diarrhoea due to inflammatory bowel disorders may not be overtly bloody

DIFFERENTIAL DIAGNOSIS

Crohn's disease

The incidence of Crohn's disease is increasing. It is an important cause of diarrhoea although, of course, numerically much less common than the irritable bowel syndrome. Diarrhoea may be due to involvement of the small bowel or colon, or both, and several pathogenic processes may cause the bowel disturbance. An understanding of these processes is important when choosing the most appropriate therapy.

Table 13.1 Differential diagnosis of chronic diarrhoea

Crohn's disease
Drugs
Malabsorption
Surgery
Endocrine causes
Irritable bowel syndrome
Ulcerative colitis
Gastrointestinal infection

Drugs

Iatrogenic causes of diarrhoea are important. Antacids, especially magnesium-containing compounds, cause diarrhoea, although perhaps this problem is becoming less common with the more liberal use of the H_2-receptor antagonists. The analgesic mefenamic acid may cause diarrhoea, as may the diuretic spironolactone. Alcohol is a very important cause of alimentary symptoms including diarrhoea; a constant alertness to the possibility of alcohol abuse should be

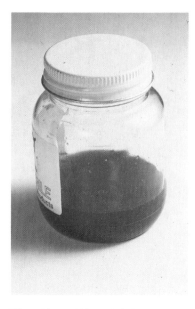

Fig. 13.1 Phenolphthalein detected in a patient's urine by the addition of alkali.

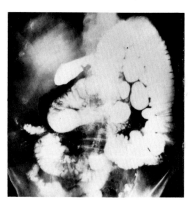

Fig. 13.2 Jejunal diverticulosis: the 'golfballs' are the diverticula.

maintained. Laxative misuse, commonly covert, may be difficult to diagnose and is frequently denied by the patient (Fig. 13.1).

Malabsorption

Malabsorption is an uncommon cause of diarrhoea, but it is an important diagnosis because effective treatment is usually possible. Pancreatic steatorrhoea may develop against a background of alcohol abuse leading to chronic pancreatitis, although this condition can also occur in the abstemious. The other main causes of pancreatic exocrine failure are carcinoma of the pancreas and cystic fibrosis. Small bowel causes of steatorrhoea include coeliac disease and bacterial overgrowth. The former is to be considered at any age, paticularly if a generalised malabsorption picture is present. Bacterial overgrowth usually develops as a consequence of a disturbed small bowel anatomy (for example jejunal diverticulosis (Fig. 13.2), a blind loop or a fistula in Crohn's disease) or abnormal motility (for example diabetes or progressive systemic sclerosis).

Surgery

Previous truncal vagotomy for peptic ulceration can lead to severe diarrhoea, although fortunately this operation is now performed less often. The combination of a vagotomy and a cholecystectomy is particularly likely to cause diarrhoea. Right hemicolectomy, especially if a significant length of terminal ileum is removed, may result in watery diarrhoea due to malabsorption of bile salts. Diarrhoea may occur after therapeutic abdominal or pelvic irradiation, which can damage the terminal ileum, again causing bile salt malabsorption.

Endocrine causes

These are uncommon, but occasionally diarrhoea may be the presenting feature of thyrotoxicosis. A gastrin-secreting tumour of the pancreas may result in recurrent and severe peptic ulceration, with diarrhoea (the Zollinger-Ellison syndrome). Other rare causes of diarrhoea include metastatic carcinoid tumour, medullary carcinoma of the thyroid, a non-beta islet-cell tumour of the pancreas and Addison's disease.

CLUES FROM THE HISTORY

It is important to determine precisely what the patient means when he complains of diarrhoea. Careful enquiry should be made as to the nature of the stool: is it hard, soft or unformed? Is there a normal stool mixed with an abnormal component such as mucus, to which the patient is referring when he speaks of diarrhoea? Is the patient experiencing a frequent call to stool but passing very little except some mucus and flatus, a feature of proctitis or ulcerative colitis? Is the patient passing a normally formed stool on some occasions and unformed stool on others? What is the frequency of visits to the lavatory to defaecate and what is the temporal pattern of these visits? Noctural diarrhoea is a good indicator of organic bowel disease and is rare in the irritable bowel syndrome. Early morning diarrhoea is a common feature of either irritable bowel syndrome or proctitis. A description of stool colour is important only when looking for the pale and greasy stool of steatorrhoea.

Urgency of defaecation may be an important clue to the presence of rectal inflammatory disease such as proctitis. Faecal incontinence should be specifically enquired about as the patient will often be too embarrassed to mention it. Incontinence may be a sign of a weakened anal sphincter, especially in the elderly parous female or the homosexual, or be a sign of rectal inflammatory bowel disease. Faecal incontinence is rare in functional bowel disorders.

> Determine precisely what the patient means when he complains of diarrhoea

The irritable bowel syndrome

The irritable bowel syndrome can be described as the cross which the gastroenterologist has to bear. It is the commonest reason for referral for a gastroenterological opinion. Its main features include abdominal pain, altered bowel habit and abdominal distension. The irritable bowel syndrome does not cause rectal bleeding and if this symptom is present an alternative explanation must be sought.

When pain is a dominant feature a previous history of abdominal surgery is not uncommon. Such operations may have been undertaken in an attempt to cure the pain and include most commonly appendicectomy, cholecystectomy, peptic ulcer surgery and occasionally hysterectomy: a testament to earlier inadequate preoperative investigation and diagnosis! It may be informative to enquire closely about the effect of any previous operation on the pain (did it help?) and about the precise surgical pathology, or lack of it, that was discovered at laparotomy. There is a high incidence of appendicectomy, resecting histologically normal appendices in patients with irritable bowel syndrome who present with right iliac fossa pain, which was inappropriately labelled as 'chronic appendicitis'.

Diarrhoea is often associated with abdominal pain (see Chapter 6). Characteristically the diarrhoea follows the pain and may relieve it. A further feature of the altered bowel habit in the irritable bowel syndrome is that there may be phases when either diarrhoea or constipation predominates. In a constipated phase, the patient may describe the stool as 'pellet-like' or like 'rabbit droppings'. Occasionally he may describe the frequent passage of such small hard stools as diarrhoea. As already indicated, the diarrhoea of a patient with irritable bowle syndrome is virtually never nocturnal; the presence of this symptom should prompt a search for an alternative diagnosis. Very occasionally the passing of mucus per rectum may be a prominent feature -- hence the old and inappropriate name of 'mucous colitis' -- but its occurrence demands the careful exclusion of organic rectal or colonic disease.

Finally it should be remembered that the shorter the history of diarrhoea, the greater the likelihood of finding an alternative diagnosis to the irritable bowel syndrome.

> Passage of mucus per rectum demands careful exclusion of organic disease

> The shorter the history of diarrhoea, the more likely a diagnosis other than irritable bowel syndrome

Crohn's disease

The combination of pain and diarrhoea may occur in Crohn's disease, particularly when this involves the small bowel. The pain is commonly colicky and related to eating; it may be due to episodes of subacute obstruction. A high-residue diet is particularly likely to exacerbate these symptoms. Vomiting may accompany such episodes of bolus colic, and easily heard borborygmi may also be present.

Alcohol

A history of heavy alcohol use may be an important clue in the patient with diarrhoea. Beer may act as a laxative and be the cause of this symptom. Of greater importance is the possibility that diarrhoea may be secondary to chronic pancreatitis, when pain is not an invariable feature. A careful enquiry about possible steatorrhoea with the characteristic pale, greasy, difficult-to-flush stool should be made.

ABNORMALITIES ON EXAMINATION

General examination

Important clues as to the cause of diarrhoea may be gained from a general examination of the patient. Evidence of weight loss should be sought and the patient should be weighed to provide a base-line for the detection of subsequent changes. Mucosal pallor as a sign of anaemia in the patient with diarrhoea may alert the physician to the presence of colitis, Crohn's disease or small bowel malabsorption. Clubbing should be sought as it occurs in disease of the small bowel, especially Crohn's disease (Fig. 13.3). Occasionally a pancreatic carcinoma will present with diarrhoea due to pancreatic duct obstruction, causing exocrine insufficiency and steatorrhoea. The presence of fever in a patient with chronic diarrhoea indicates that inflammatory bowel disease is the most likely cause. The smell of alcohol on the breath is an important physical sign, especially during a morning consultation. Signs of thyrotoxicosis should be sought, particularly if the diarrhoea is associated with marked weight loss (Fig. 13.4).

Neurotic features are sometimes prominent in the patient with nervous diarrhoea, and bitten nails and a patient's general demeanour may be important clues, although it is salutary to remember that their presence does not exclude organic causes of diarrhoea.

Fig. 13.3   Finger-clubbing may reveal small intestinal disease.

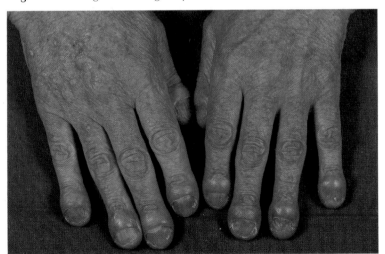

Fig. 13.4   Thyrotoxicosis causing diarrhoea, confirmed by a thyroid scan.

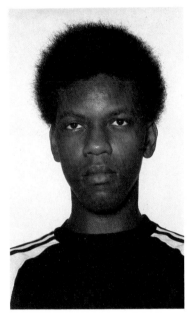

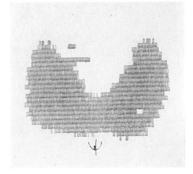

Raynaud's phenomenon (Fig. 13.5) and other cutaneous features of progressive systemic sclerosis may suggest involvement of the gut in the same pathological process and explain the origin of an otherwise obscure diarrhoea.

Oedema in the patient with diarrhoea (Fig. 13.6) may be due to hypoalbuminaemia secondary to malabsorption or gastrointestinal protein loss.

Examination of the systems

Abdominal examination may be disappointingly uninformative in the patient with diarrhoea. 'Erythema ab igne' from a comforting hot water bottle (Fig. 13.7) may testify to the longevity of pain and if associated with diarrhoea may suggest chronic pancreatitis as a cause. More rarely, chronic intestinal ischaemia may be the explanation of this combination. It is said that a hot water bottle mark is more likely to occur with organic disease, but exceptions occur. Careful abdominal inspection, particularly in the slim patient, may reveal an intra-abdominal mass.

Tenderness is a frequent sign in the patient with the irritable bowel syndrome. This may be elicited at any site and it often occurs in one or both iliac fossae. A palpable descending colon is another common finding in this condition. A mass, particularly in the right iliac fossa, may point strongly towards the possibility of Crohn's disease in the patient with diarrhoea.

Rectal examination must be preceded by careful inspection of the perianal region with good illumination, taking care to

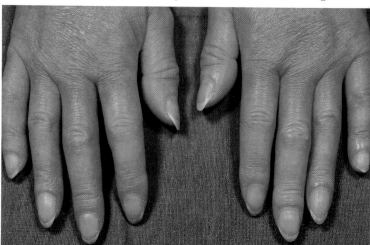

Fig. 13.5 Scleroderma of the fingers with calcinosis cutis and Raynaud's phenomenon.

spread the anal margins to look for a fissure or other local pathology (see Chapter 19). Too often this part of the examination becomes a hasty glance in poor light before the digital examination. Anal and perianal lesions are particularly common in Crohn's disease, especially when this involves the large bowel. If a fissure is present, digital examination must be carried out using a local anaesthetic gel as a lubricant. A deformed anal canal may be a further clue to Crohn's disease, and the presence of blood will be an indication of the need for further investigation.

A most important part of the physical examination of the patient with chronic diarrhoea, and one which is often very informative, is proctosigmoidoscopy. There is no reason why the lower rectal mucosa cannot be examined by the general practitioner in the surgery. Cheap disposable plastic proctoscopes are readily available and proctoscopy in the surgery may alert the physician to the presence of colitis. Visualisation of a normal rectal mucosa effectively excludes proctitis or proctosigmoiditis in the majority of patients, although occasionally a normal rectum does occur in the patient with ulcerative colitis. A normal rectal mucosa does not exclude a diagnosis of Crohn's disease of the colon. In the full assessment of a patient with diarrhoea a rectal biopsy will be taken even if the rectum and lower sigmoid look normal, as there may be histological pointers to the presence of colitis.

Fig. 13.6 Ankle oedema due to hypoalbuminaemia in a young patient.

Fig. 13.7 An abdominal hot water bottle mark.

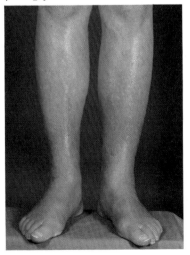

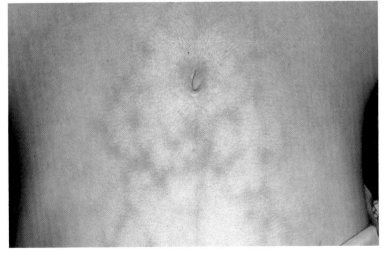

Examination of the patient with diarrhoea is incomplete without careful inspection of the stool. This may be achieved during sigmoidoscopy or on the gloved finger after the rectal examination. Much can be learned: rock-hard faeces may cause impaction with spurious diarrhoea; an unformed bloody stool indicates the presence of a colitis; the fat-laden stool of the patient with steatorrhoea is usually unmistakable.

INVESTIGATIONS

In some patients a confident clinical diagnosis of irritable bowel syndrome will be possible and investigation will be unnecessary. In other patients the choice of investigation will depend upon the range of differential diagnoses being entertained.

Haematology

A full blood count and ESR may provide important clues, any abnormality making the diagnosis of irritable bowel syndrome untenable (see Chapter 16). In the patient with inflammatory bowel disease a raised ESR may occur, although a normal sedimentation rate does not exclude Crohn's disease or colitis. Anaemia is common in the inflammatory bowel diseases and disorders of small bowel absorption, but is unusual in pancreatic steatorrhoea. Macrocytosis may be an important clue to alcohol abuse or the presence of folate deficiency. Identification of Howell-Jolly bodies in the blood film will suggest hyposplenism and, in the presence of chronic diarrhoea, this will point to a diagnosis of either coeliac disease or ulcerative colitis.

Biochemistry

The serum albumin is often decreased in Crohn's disease and coeliac disease. Biochemical screening may reveal evidence of malabsorption with a low calcium, raised alkaline phosphatase, low vitamin D and prolonged prothrombin time. Steatorrhoea has to be quantified by a three-day collection of faeces, whilst the patient takes a diet containing fat. A carton of single cream taken every day of the collection is usually sufficient provoke steatorrhoea in a susceptible patient.

Direct tests of absorption can be helpful in suspected small bowel disease. The xylose tolerance test is often abnormal in coeliac disease or extensive small intestinal Crohn's disease.

The role of the lactose tolerance test is still disputed: failure of the blood glucose concentration to rise after oral lactose (the disaccharide of glucose and galactose) indicates deficiency of the enzyme lactase. If the test is associated with diarrhoea, abdominal cramps and bloating, this indicates true lactose intolerance. In such patients a reduced lactose ('milk-free') diet may produce symptomatic benefit. Alactasia may occur in coeliac disease, as an association in a small proportion of patients with colitis or as a transient phenomenon after an acute gastroenteritis. It may also occur in normal people and is especially common in those with genetic roots from outside Western Europe.

Stool tests for occult blood may also sometimes be helpful in a patient with chronic diarrhoea. The presence of repeatedly positive occult blood tests in this context indicates a possible colitis, colonic carcinoma or polyp.

Microbiology

Infective causes of chronic diarrhoea are uncommon. However, giardiasis or amoebiasis should not be forgotten, especially in the patient who has travelled abroad. Leningrad and Asia, Africa and South America are all areas with endemic giardiasis. Although there is usually a sudden onset of symptoms in giardiasis, the disorder may present insidiously. Stool examination is not always positive in either condition: two or even three samples may need to be examined. Occasionally giardiasis may only be confirmed by examination of a duodenal aspirate or biopsy. Serological tests for amoebiasis are positive in a helpful proportion of cases, especially if there is an associated liver abscess. Amoebae may be identified in a rectal biopsy.

Radiology

PLAIN ABDOMINAL X-RAY. This examination is of value in the differential diagnosis of chronic diarrhoea by identifying pancreatic calcification which may be present in some patients with chronic pancreatitis (Fig. 13.8). Thus if the patient has a history of alcohol abuse, and complains of diarrhoea, especially if this is suggestive of steatorrhoea, then a plain abdominal X-ray may be very informative. The absence of calcification

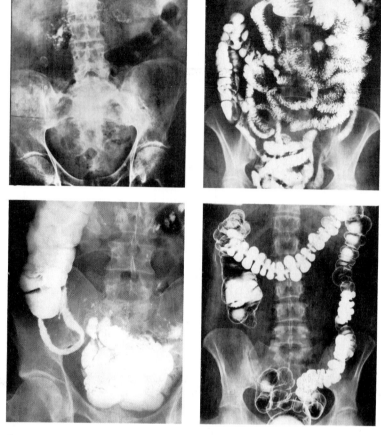

Fig. 13.8 Pancreatic calcification. A large calculus in the head of the pancreas and diffuse calcification in the head, body and tail of the pancreas.

Fig. 13.9 Barium follow-through of a normal small intestine.

Fig. 13.10 Crohn's disease of the terminal ileum.

Fig. 13.11 Spasm due to irritable bowel, shown on a barium enema.

does not, however, exclude pancreatic exocrine insufficiency as a cause of diarrhoea.

BARIUM STUDIES. The conventional barium meal is not often helpful in investigating the cause of chronic diarrhoea, except in the rare patient with a gastrocolic fistula which is usually due to a carcinoma (stomach or colon) or chronic gastric ulcer.

Small bowel radiology, with a conventional barium meal and follow-through (Fig. 13.9), or the more recently introduced small bowel enema, is the more appropriate investigation in a patient with diarrhoea. This may confirm a suspected diagnosis of Crohn's disease (Fig. 13.10), or allow identification of jejunal diverticulosis, or the intestinal manifestations of progressive systemic sclerosis. An isolated duodenal diverticulum is a common finding and is rarely, if ever, the cause of diarrhoea. If steatorrhoea is present, then small bowel radiology is indicated if a pancreatic cause is not present; a barium enema is an inappropriate investigation of steatorrhoea.

A barium enema is essential if sigmoidoscopy has demonstrated features of a colitis, once infective causes have been excluded. Changes of ulcerative or Crohn's colitis may be revealed (see Chapter 15). A carcinoma of the colon may be demonstrated and it is an important cause of diarrhoea, even in the absence of rectal bleeding or positive occult blood. In the patient with irritable bowel syndrome areas of spasm may be demonstrated (Fig. 13.11); showing these X-rays to the patient may be a helpful adjunct when explaining the disorder of motility in this condition.

WHICH PATIENT TO X-RAY. Clearly if rectal bleeding accompanies the diarrhoea then a barium enema is indicated. This should, of course, be preceeded by rectal examination and proctosigmoidoscopy. In the older patient, in whom the chances of finding significant colonic pathology are higher, especially if the passage of mucus per rectum is a feature, again radiology of the lower bowel is warranted.

If anaemia accompanies diarrhoea, radiology will probably be necessary, but it may be difficult to decide which end of the alimentary tract to investigate first, if other clues are not present. In the absence of dyspepsia, a barium enema is probably the first choice. In the younger patient the choice of X-ray will depend upon which differential diagnoses are being considered: if malabsorption due to either coeliac disease or Crohn's disease is considered likely then small bowel radiology would be appropriate.

In many patients with chronic diarrhoea due to the irritable bowel syndrome radiology will be unnecessary if a confident clinical diagnosis can be made.

Colonoscopy

In the patient with chronic diarrhoea colonoscopy may show definite features of a colitis even when a good quality double-contrast barium enema is considered normal. Colonoscopy is indicated if there is a strong clinical suspicion of inflammatory bowel disease, especially if there is no abnormality on sigmoidoscopy or rectal biopsy (Fig. 13.12). With this

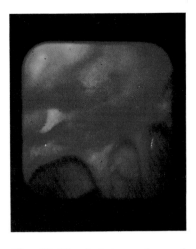

Fig. 13.12   Aphthous ulcers of Crohn's disease.

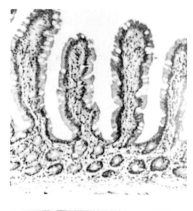

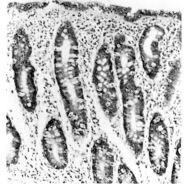

Fig. 13.13   Healthy jejunal mucosa showing normal villi.

Fig. 13.14   Subtotal villus atrophy in coelic disease. Note the absence of villi.

technique the whole of the colon can be inspected and mucosal biopsies taken for histological examination. It is sometimes possible to examine the terminal ileum; this may be provide histological proof, confirming a clinical diagnosis of Crohn's disease.

Another diagnostically helpful clue, which may be demonstrated by colonoscopy, is the detection of melanosis coli. This is a darkening of the colonic mucosa due to accumulation of pigment, occurring as a consequence of long-term use of anthraquinone laxatives such as senna or cascara. It must be emphasised that the detection of melanosis coli is only a marker of previous long-term use of laxatives and as such is quite common. The presence of melanosis coli does not necessarily mean that the patient's diarrhoea is due to laxative abuse.

Rare patients, who secretly abuse laxatives, present with profound diarrhoea, and often muscle weakness due to hypokalaemia; they deny laxative ingestion. A high index of suspicion is required to make this diagnosis. Some laxatives can be detected in the urine or faeces, but the patient's belongings may have to be searched. Such patients usually have a psychiatric illness.

Jejunal biopsy

The diagnosis of coeliac disease can only be made with certainty by jejunal biopsy. The finding of an atrophic mucosa without villi, presenting the picture of subtotal villous atrophy, confirms the diagnosis (Figs 13.13, 13.14). Other rarer causes of diarrhoea may also be diagnosed by jejunal biopsy and these include Whipple's disease, intestinal lymphangiectasia and small intestinal lymphoma.

Pancreatic function tests

Urine testing for glucose is the simplest pancreatic function test and should not be forgotten. Whatever the result, this should be followed by a random blood sugar estimation and a glucose tolerance test may be needed to detect mild endocrine pancreatic failure.

If steatorrhoea is present then tests may be needed to exclude pancreatic insufficiency. Currently the only proven function tests require duodenal intubation and collection of pancreatic secretions. The simplest and most widely available is the

Lundh test. In this test the trypsin content of the duodenal aspirate is measured following stimulation by a standard test meal. If steatorrhoea is due to exocrine pancreatic insufficiency, tryptic activity is usually reduced.

Disease of the pancreas, sufficient to cause exocrine deficiency, can usually be demonstrated by endoscopic retrograde cholangiopancreatography (ERCP), when the endoscopist threads a cannula through the ampulla of Vater into the pancreatic duct, which is then outlined by radio-opaque dye (Fig. 13.15).

Other investigations

Additional tests will be needed to elucidate the rarer causes of chronic diarrhoea: thyroid function tests to exclude thyrotoxicosis; urinary 5-HIAA measurement for suspected carcinoid; fasting plasma gastrin for the Zollinger-Ellison syndrome; and vasoactive intestinal polypeptide for the extremely rare pancreatic cholera or the WDHA syndrome.

MANAGEMENT

Irritable bowel syndrome

Management of the patient with the irritable bowel syndrome begins with making the diagnosis. Whenever possible, and this

Fig. 13.15 Chronic pancreatitis revealed by retrograde pancreatography, compared to the normal appearance.

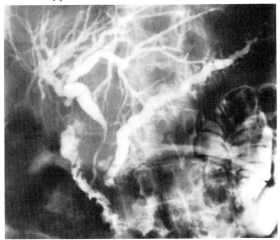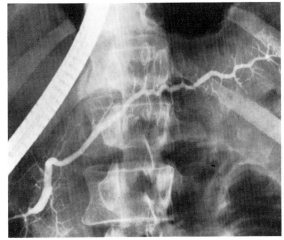

will prove to be the case in the majority of patients, a positive diagnosis should be made rather than one of exclusion. This positive approach will be conveyed to the patient, giving greater confidence in subsequent management. An approach to the patient which begins by indicating that all tests are negative, and therefore there is nothing wrong, is to be deprecated. On the contrary it is important to indicate that you do know what is wrong with the patient and that any negative tests are simply serving to exclude possible alternatives. Such an approach is particularly important with the patient who has had multiple investigations, possibly in many different hospital departments, even unhelpful surgery. Tell the patient that you know what is wrong and give it a name.

The all-encompassing term 'irritable bowel syndrome' is useful because it does not pretend to indicate an aetiology, it does not erroneously refer to 'colitis', and it does not implicate any particular part of the gastrointestinal tract. Moreover it is a name easily remembered by the patient. A 'take-home' diagnostic label is important for the patient and is better than a bland 'there is nothing wrong'.

The patient should be told in a positive way that the condition does not develop into anything more serious. Tell the patient that it is nothing to do with cancer or colitis, which are the two commonest fears.

It is advisable to attempt to explain to the patient the mechanism of production of the symptoms in by the irritable bowel syndrome. This is limited to a certain extent by our own lack of understanding of pathophysiology. Explanation, of course, must be tailored to suit the patient's level of intelligence and knowledge of biology. In this context I find invaluable a quick sketch of the gastrointestinal tract which the patient can keep. Indicating that the gut is a long hollow tube, like a bicycle tyre inner-tube, with muscle in its wall, is a good starting point. Diarrhoea can then be explained as muscle over-activity, constipation as inactivity, pain as muscle spasm and windy distension as air trapping in the bowel between two areas of spasm. Although this is clearly at variance with what is known about the disordered motility of the condition it has the merit of simplicity and of being understood by the patient.

Diarrhoea due to the irritable bowel syndrome can often be improved with anti-diarrhoeals. Loperamide is a useful potent anti-diarrhoeal without central side effects. The patient should be instructed to be flexible with the dose and one to three 2 mg capsules daily are usually sufficient to improve stool frequency.

Tell the patient that you know what is wrong and give it a name

Two capsules on retiring may be helpful to the patient with
early morning diarrhoea. Codeine phosphate and Lomotil are
effective alternatives, but they may cause fatal respiratory
depression if taken in error by small children.

The use of bulking agents may lessen diarrhoea. The fibre
content of bran helps because of its water-holding properties.
Proprietary forms of bulk-forming agents are numerous.
Occasionally diarrhoea and flatus may be aggravated by a
high-fibre diet; this may respond to a reduction of dose, but is
may necessitate discontinuation of the roughage.

Crohn's disease

Diarrhoea due to Crohn's disease has many causes which in
turn influence management. Diarrhoea due to Crohn's colitis
is discussed in Chapter 15.

Increased bowel frequency due to small bowel Crohn's
disease may respond to antidiarrhoeals, such as loperamide 2
mg three times daily, tailoring the dose to suit the patient. If
there is any question of narrowing of the small bowel due to
Crohn's disease, as might be suggested by the presence of
colicky pain after food, bulking agents are positively
contraindicated. Such patients may get episodes of colicky
pain, relieved by diarrhoea, due to subacute bolus obstruction
of the small intestine. Such patients often respond to a
'stricture' diet which excludes lumps of food residue, such as
sweetcorn, orange segments or cabbage stalks.

Oral steroids usually reduce small bowel diarrhoea due to
active Crohn's disease. Bacterial overgrowth in the small bowel
may cause diarrhoea and this tends to occur particularly when
there is a stenosing lesion or after an ileocolic anastomosis.
Oral metronidazole, tetracycline or lincomycin may be helpful
in this situation, and repeated short courses of antibiotic may
be necessary. When diarrhoea arises because of terminal ileal
disease, with failure of bile salt reabsorption (bile salt induced
diarrhoea), cholestyramine (one to two sachets three times
daily) may be helpful, although some patients find this
medication unpalatable.

Pancreatic malabsorption

This is treated with pancreatic enzyme supplements, whose
efficacy may be enhanced by concurrent administration of
cimetidine to reduce the gastric acid secretion that destroys

pancreatic enzyme activity. A low fat diet is usually helpful if adequate control is not achieved using pancreatic supplements.

Coeliac disease

This condition requires a strict and life-long gluten-free diet, initiated with the help of a dietician. Relapses are most commonly due to dietary indiscretion. Membership of the Coeliac Society (P.O. Box 181, London NW2) should be recommended to all patients, as the Society keeps an up-to-date register or proprietary foods, recording the presence or absence of gluten. At the initiation of treatment, when multiple deficiencies may be present, supplements with iron, folic acid, calcium, potassium, magnesium, vitamin D or vitamin K may be necessary. Gluten-free foods can be prescribed on the standard FP10 form which should be marked 'ACBS' (Advisory Committee on Borderline Substances).

FURTHER READING

Cooke WT, Mallas E, Prior P, Allan RN (1980) Crohn's disease: course, treatment and long-term prognosis. Quart J Med 195: 363-384.

Kirsner JB, Shorter RG (1982) Recent developments in 'nonspecific' inflammatory bowel disease. N Engl J Med 306: 775-786, 837-848.

Lennard-Jones JE (1983) Functional gastrointestinal disorders. N Engl J Med 308: 431-435.

Review Article (1983) Irritable bowel syndrome and its treatment. Drug Ther Bull 21: 37-39.

Thompson WG, Heaton KW (1980) Functional bowel disorders in apparently healthy people. Gastroenterology 79: 283-288.

Welch CE, Malt RA (1983) Abdominal surgery, part 1. N Engl J Med 308: 624-632.

Doctor, I'm allergic to food

Food allergy is much in the public eye. There have been many popular books and magazine articles linking food with a wide range of symptoms, some of which are gastrointestinal. Patients often attribute an unacceptable bowel habit or abdominal discomfort to food allergy.

The concept of food allergy was introduced in the United States in the first part of this century. It was slow to cross the Atlantic, gaining a hold in Great Britain only in the last decade. In the meantime some specific gut diseases had been objectively linked with particular foods (e.g. coeliac disease with gluten and hypolactasia with milk) but scepticism had grown up amongst medical scientists against the vague and woolly claims of the food allergists that virtually any disease could be caused by any food. Thus it is an area about which British doctors tend to be ill-informed.

Gut symptoms may be linked to foods by a number of mechanisms. These include true food allergy, specific pharmacological reactions to food constituents and food intolerances.

True *food allergies* (Fig. 14.1) involve a Type I or Type III hypersensitivity reaction; they are associated with raised serum IgE, circulating immune complexes and eosinophilia. The symptoms, which often include systemic manifestations such as urticarial rashes and gut symptoms, come on about 20 minutes after the ingestion of the food. Soothill has indicated those symptoms which may be securely ascribed to food allergy (Table 14.1). The incidence of food allergy is higher amongst atopic individuals than amongst the general population.

Food idiosyncrasies may be manifested either as a result of an enzyme deficiency or as a result of the pharmacological action of molecules contained in the foods. Hypolactasia has already been mentioned: many adults cannot tolerate the milk sugar lactose, as they have a deficit of the disaccharidase lactase that digests the sugar. Phenylketonuria is a much rarer condition caused by an inborn error of metabolism: an enzyme deficiency

British doctors tend to be ill-informed about food allergy

Table 14.1 Symptoms securely ascribed to allergy (Soothill)

General
Sudden death
Anaphylaxis

Alimentary
Vomiting
Abdominal pain
 and distension } in children
Diarrhoea

Skin
Urticaria
Angioneurotic oedema
Eczema

Respiratory
Rhinitis
Asthma

General (secondary to gut allergy)
Failure to thrive
Anaemia (iron loss)
Oedema (protein loss)

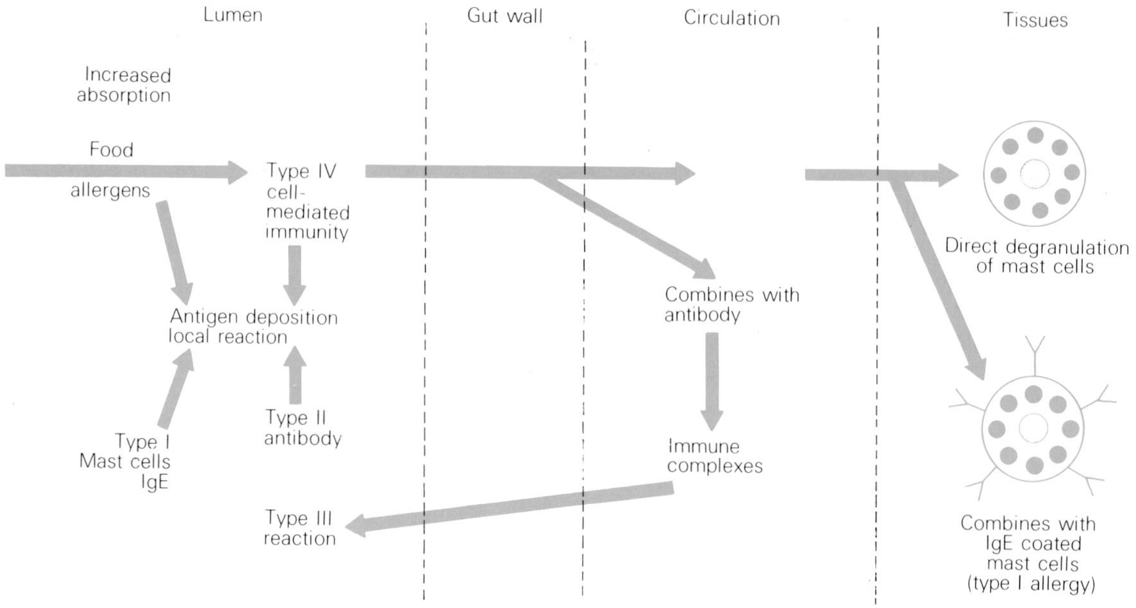

Fig. 14.1 Mechanisms of food allergy.

Many patients with irritable bowel syndrome may suffer from food intolerance

allows dietary phenylalanine to accumulate in the body causing progressive damage. The caffeine in coffee has a number of pharmacological actions: it can give rise to palpitations and increases heartburn in susceptible individuals.

Most *food intolerances* are mediated by other, as yet unclear, mechanisms, although there is some evidence that large bowel prostaglandin production may be important (Fig. 14.2). No immunological mechanisms have so far been detected. The symptoms due to food intolerance come on any time from 1 to 48 hours after ingestion of a food, and they mainly involve abdominal pain and diarrhoea. Systemic symptoms are usually non-specific: general weariness, headache and muscular aches and pains. There is no association between food intolerance and atopy. A high proportion of patients with the irritable bowel syndrome may suffer from food intolerance.

DIFFERENTIAL DIAGNOSIS

The differential diagnosis of any patient with abdominal pain and diarrhoea is extremely wide (see Chapters 6 and 13), but it is summarised in Table 14.2.

CLUES FROM THE HISTORY

Irritable bowel syndrome due to food intolerance is an extremely common disease; it is most prevalent amongst women aged 20-40. Clear-cut cases are easy to sort out. If symptoms are caused by either seasonal foods or exotic or expensive foods which the patient eats rarely, the link between food and symptom is easy to see. Indeed, the patient may simply seek reassurance that such a phenomenon is recognised, having already decided that she will avoid the food in future. Alternatively, she may enquire whether there is anything which will allow her to eat the food with impunity.

Unfortunately the majority of intolerances involve very common foods. It is unusual for patients to connect chronic symptoms with everyday foods, and so dietary histories are futile. Indeed, most patients with irritable bowel syndrome do not appreciate that they have a food intolerance at all. However, the history will produce helpful pointers towards the identification of these patients who may benefit from trying a diet.

Most intolerances involve very common foods and dietary histories are futile

Abdominal pain, with diarrhoea or alternating periods of diarrhoea and constipation, is frequent. The pain is usually low and central or felt in one or both iliac fossae. Care must be taken to distinguish the pain of food intolerance from abdominal pain due to a musculoskeletal cause, which is also particularly common in women of this age. However, if the pain is associated with bowel actions, relieved by defaecation rather than by a night's sleep on a firm bed, and not aggravated by physical activity, it is reasonable to ascribe it to the gut.

The diarrhoea of food intolerance commonly occurs on awakening in the morning, leaving the rest of the day relatively free of trouble. Food intolerance does not cause nocturnal diarrhoea or rectal bleeding.

Food intolerance does not cause nocturnal diarrhoea or rectal bleeding

Table 14.2 Principal differential diagnoses to be excluded in patients suspected of having food intolerance

Symptoms of diarrhoea	*Symptoms of lower abdominal pain*
Infective	Cancer of the colon
Ulcerative colitis	Crohn's disease
Crohn's disease	Gynaecological problems
Cancer of the colon	Musculoskeletal problems
Malabsorption	

Table 14.3   Analysis of symptoms in 89 patients with food intolerance

Abdominal pain	73%
Diarrhoea	61%
Weariness	52%
Headache	38%
Migraine	11%
Fluid retention	27%
Constipation	23%
Abdominal distension	21%

Sigmoidoscopy should be used to exclude more serious disease

Various additional non-specific symptoms may be associated with food intolerance, headache and weariness being particularly common (Table 14.3). Almost 50% of our patients connect the onset of their symptoms with a gut infection, a course of antibiotics or gynaecological or abdominal surgery. These precipitants are worth enquiring for. Many patients observe that gut symptoms vary with their menstrual cycle with a predictable pattern.

ABNORMALITIES ON EXAMINATION

The role of physical examination in these patients is to exclude more serious conditions. Abdominal examination often reveals palpable, somewhat tender, ascending or descending colon, but the presence of an abdominal mass or palpable liver suggests that food intolerance is not the diagnosis. Sigmoidoscopy should always be performed to exclude more serious disease; rectal bleeding is not due to food intolerance.

INVESTIGATIONS

The investigation of patients suspected of having food intolerance is aimed at excluding other diseases, as there is as yet no diagnostic test for the condition. Blood screening tests should include: a full blood count including ESR, liver function tests and urea and electrolytes. Estimation of an acute-phase protein (C-reactive protein or orosomucoid) will screen for Crohn's disease. A stool culture should be performed, faecal fats measured and occult blood sought. If all these tests are normal, it is safe to assume that the diarrhoea is unlikely to be due to infection, malabsorption or neoplasia, but it is wise to perform a barium enema in patients over the age of 40.

Specific tests to identify the foods which upset the patient have been disappointing. Skin testing using food extracts is unreliable. Intradermal tests are said to be better than prick testing, but when we studied double-blind intradermal skin tests in six patients whose food intolerances were well established, the accuracy of identification of the foods which provoked their symptoms was only 53%. Radio-allergosorbent (RAST) testing, which tests for IgE reactive to specific allergens, is also unreliable; serum IgE and circulating immune complex levels are normal.

MANAGEMENT

Dietary manipulation

A trial of a fortnight's high-fibre diet should be made, as it will help a few, but the most effective treatment for most patients with food intolerance is a diet which allows the foods which cause symptoms in each individual to be identified, so that they can be avoided subsequently. Elimination dieting is a way of achieving this: the patient is instructed to limit the diet to one meat, one fruit and spring water for five to eight days. When this leads to a complete remission of symptoms, one food is re-introduced at a time, watching for those which provoke symptoms.

Elimination dieting is considerably more easily described than done; we have now stopped using this technique, as we found it too difficult and too unpleasant for our patients. However, analysis of the foods provoking symptoms in 80 patients who had successfully followed an elimination diet under our care allowed the design of a new exclusion diet (Table 14.4). Using this dietary regimen patients avoid all the foods which were found to provoke symptoms in more than 20% of our original patients (Table 14.5). It is possible, of course, that even the foods allowed by the exclusion diet may also provoke their symptoms, but if the patients keep to the diet and record the timing of all foods eaten in relation to symptoms, it may be possible to spot the offenders.

We have stopped using elimination dieting

After two weeks on the exclusion diet, when all symptoms have cleared, the excluded foods are re-introduced one by one; those that do not provoke symptoms are added to the basic diet. When all testing is finished, the final diet should be checked for nutritional adequacy. Our patients have tended to require supplements of calcium, iron and vitamin C. Jejunal biopsy should be performed in wheat-intolerant patients to exclude coeliac disease.

If a patient is not fully recovered after two weeks on an exclusion diet, it is not worth persisting with a dietary approach. Continued food restriction is extremely irksome. Those patients who have multiple food intolerances are best treated symptomatically to avoid the development of an obsessional fixation on dietary manoeuvres.

Many patients find that after some months on their diet the food intolerances disappear. We suggest that patients should retest foods at yearly intervals and eat foods freely when they no longer provoke symptoms.

Retest foods at yearly intervals

Table 14.4   The exclusion diet for patients with gastrointestinal symptoms

	Not allowed	*Allowed*
Meat	Preserved meats Bacon Sausages	All other meats
Fish	Smoked fish Shellfish	White fish
Vegetables	Potatoes Onions	All other vegetables/salads Pulses (peas, beans, lentils)
Fruits	Citrus fruits (oranges, grapefruit, lemons)	All other fruits (apples, bananas, pears)
Cereals	Wheat (e.g. bread, cakes, biscuits, pasta, noodles, semolina, breakfast cereals such as Weetabix, Shredded Wheat Rye (e.g. crispbreads) Barley Corn (e.g. cornflakes, tinned foods, gravy browning, custard powder, cornflour	Rice, including ground rice and rice flour Rice Krispies Rice cakes Sago Millet* Buckwheat* Tapioca
Cooking oil	Corn oil Vegetable oil	Sunflower oil Safflower oil Soya oil Olive oil

Dietary restrictions may dismay patients. Clinical ecologists claim that it is possible to desensitise the patients by the sublingual or subcutaneous administration of dilute food extracts. We are currently conducting a double-blind trial of the technique, and while it would be wrong to prejudge the result it is nevertheless our experience that patients with gastrointestinal food intolerance rarely benefit from this procedure. At present there would seem to be little justification for referring such patients to a clinical ecologist.

Drug treatment

Some drugs also have roles to play in helping food-intolerant patients. Sodium cromoglycate seems useful in allowing patients established on a diet to stray from it on those social

	Not allowed	*Allowed*
Dairy products	Cow's milk including dried milk such as Marvel	Goat's milk* Soya milk
	Butter	
	Margarine, other than	Tomor kosher margarine Sainsbury's Low-Fat Spread
	Yoghurt, other than	Goat's milk yoghurt*
	Cheese, other than	Goat's milk cheese*
	Eggs	
Beverages	Tea, other than	Herbal tea such as camomile
	Coffee, beans, instant or decaffeinated	
	Fruit squashes	
	Fresh orange or grapefruit juice	Other fresh juices, e.g. apple, pineapple, tomato
	Alcohol	
Miscellaneous	Yeast, yeast extract or Marmite	Sea salt
	Preservatives	Herbs
	Chocolate	Spices, in moderation
	Nuts	Sugar
		Honey

This diet excludes all those foods which are most likely to cause food intolerance. Foods should all be fresh or frozen; tinned or packet food should not be allowed as it is important that food preservatives should be avoided. Items marked * are generally available from healthfood shops.

This diet should be followed for at least two weeks.

occasions when they will be unable to control what they eat. Four to six capsules, opened and dissolved in a small quantity of very hot water with extra cool water then added, should be swilled around the mouth and swallowed 20 minutes before the meal and then again immediately before it. This technique should not be used more frequently then once every 10 days, as frequent use appears to increase food intolerance. The mechanism of action of sodium cromoglycate in these patients is unclear.

Ibuprofen 400 mg three times a day may be tried in patients who lack the insight and determination required to establish

Table 14.5   Foods found to provoke symptoms in patients with food intolerance

Wheat	65%
Corn	37%
Dairy products	37%
Coffee	32%
Oats	31%
Rye	28%
Eggs	28%
Tea	27%
Barley	25%
Potatoes	25%
Citrus fruit	24%
Preservatives	23%
Chocolate	20%
Onions	20%

and maintain a diet which avoids symptoms. It blocks the production of 2-series prostaglandins from arachidonic acid (Fig. 14.2). Propranolol (40 mg three times a day) and amitryptyline (25 mg at night) can also be useful in this group of patients, as they block the peripheral effects of prostaglandins. It is to be expected that corticosteroids would also be effective, but it would be most difficult to justify their use in a relatively benign condition.

TRUE FOOD ALLERGY

True food allergy is a phenomenon which is rarely seen in adults. It is much rarer than food intolerance. It can be seen in babies who develop cow's milk allergy. In this condition, susceptible babies up to the age of 18-24 months develop diarrhoea and an urticarial rash, particularly if the milk is spilled on the skin, in a matter of minutes after exposure to cow's milk. The Type I hypersensitivity response may be so severe as to cause anaphylactic collapse, and has been implicated as a cause of cot death when milk proteins are

---

Sample menu for a patient on the exclusion diet

Breakfast	Buckwheat porridge, made by adding dried fruit to cooked buckwheat, *or*
	Rice Krispies with goat's or soya milk
	Apple juice
	Sago crispbreads
Lunch	Meat or fish
	Rice
	Vegetables or salad
	Fruit *or* milk pudding using goat's or soya milk
Supper	Meat or fish
	Millet
	Vegetables or salad
	Fruit *or* goat's milk yoghurt

Biscuits, pastry, crumbles, etc. can be made using rice, sago and soya flours, which are available from healthfood shops

Re-introduction of foods after the exclusion diet

When symptoms have cleared foods may be re-introduced in the order shown below. *Each food should be tested for two days.* If your symptoms do not recur you may assume that the introduced food was safe and go on to add another food. This food can now be included in any subsequent meal. If your symptoms did recur, then the new food was probably responsible and it should be omitted from your diet in future.

If a reaction occurs, it will usually last for two or three days, but may go on longer. During this time it is impossible to assess your reaction to other foods, so stick to foods you already know to be safe. *Do not introduce any new foods until you are well again.* A mixture of 2 teaspoons of sodium bicarbonate in half a pint of water will help to reduce the duration of the reaction.

You must keep a diary of all the foods you eat and any symptoms which occur in any part of the day.

Introduce foods in this order:

Potatoes
Milk
Yeast (take 3 brewer's yeast tablets or 2 tablespoons
  of baker's yeast in water)
Tea
Rye (try Ryvita or rye bread which contains no wheat flour,
  but test bread only if yeast was negative)
Butter
Onions
Eggs
Oats
Coffee (test coffee beans and instant coffee)
Chocolate (test plain chocolate, not milk)
Barley
Citrus fruits
Corn (test cornflour or corn on the cob)
Cheese
White wine
Shellfish
Yoghurt
Wheat (test wholemeal bread)
Nuts
Preservatives (e.g. fruit squashes, tinned foods, sausages,
  smoked fish)

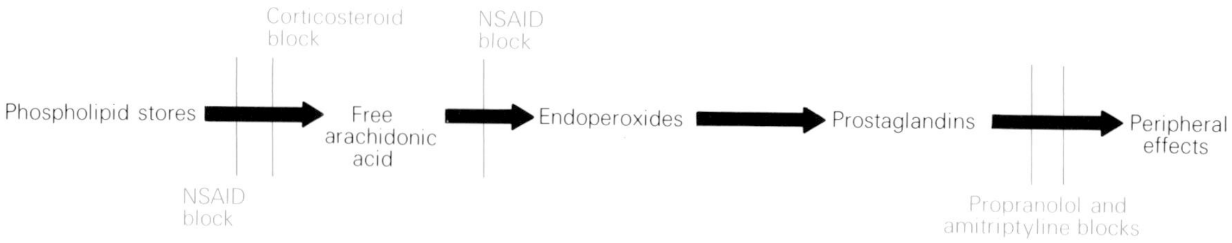

Fig. 14.2 Production of series 2 prostaglandins and the effect of drugs on the process.

inhaled. Sufferers are often born into atopic families, are eczematous and may be unhealthy despite reaching developmental milestones at the normal rate. Serum IgE may be raised but this is not significant if there are other signs of atopy. Jejunal biopsy shows a flat mucosa while the child is receiving cow's milk. Infants with cow's milk allergy should be breast-fed or given a suitable bottle mixture (e.g. Prosobee before six months and Nutramigen after six months of age). The extremely rare older child or adult with true food allergy may be managed either by excluding the offending food from the diet or by the regular use of sodium cromoglycate as previously described.

FURTHER READING

Alun Jones V, McLaughlan P, Shorthouse M, Workman, E, Hunter JO (1982) Food intolerance: a major factor in the pathogenesis of irritable bowel syndrome. Lancet 3: 1115-1117.

Boothby CB (1981) Management of gastrointestinal allergy in childhood. Update 943-995.

Coombs RRA (1980) Proceedings of the First Food Allergy Workshop. London: Medicare.

Lessof MH, Wraith DG, Merritt TG, Merritt J, Buisseret PD (1980) Food allergy and intolerance in 100 patients - local and systemic effects. Q Jl Med NS 195: 259-271.

Pearson DJ, Rix KJB, Bentley SJ (1983) Food allergy: how much in the mind? Lancet 1: 1259-1261.

Soothill JF (1981) Food allergy. In: Pepys J, Edwards AM (eds): The Mast Cell: Its Role in Health and Disease. London: Pitman Medical, 367-370.

Doctor, I've bloody diarrhoea

15

The appearance of blood in the motions inevitably causes a degree of alarm to the sufferer. It should suggest to his general practitioner that significant gastrointestinal disease is present and that urgent investigation is necessary.

Some of the disorders which cause bloody diarrhoea are self-limiting and often need little in the way of specific therapy. Others may cause serious ill-health and frequently require detailed investigation and specialised treatment.

The key factor in sorting out what is going on is to get to grips with the problem rapidly. Much of the morbidity (and possibly the mortality) in some of the conditions to be discussed can be attributed to undue delay in initiating appropriate tests.

DIFFERENTIAL DIAGNOSIS

Patients who pass loose motions containing blood may have developed any one of a large variety of conditions, some common and others much less so. The range of possibilities is listed in Table 15.1.

Bacterial infections

SALMONELLA. About 10,000 cases of salmonellosis are reported to the Public Health Laboratory Service in England and Wales each year. The most common isolate is *Salmonella typhimurium,* although a wide variety of curious serotypes are now recognised. After an incubation period of 12 to 24 hours, the patient typically presents with an acute gastroenteritis. Diarrhoea, vomiting and abdominal pain are the predominant symptoms, and about a third of patients have frank blood in the motions. The illness usually lasts only a few days, and systemic dissemination of the infection is uncommon. It should be remembered that diarrhoea and bleeding are relatively late

Table 15.1 Differential diagnosis of bloody diarrhoea

Infections and infestations
Salmonellosis
(Enteric tuberculosis)
Shigellosis
(Gonococcal proctitis)
Campylobacter
Pseudomembranous colitis
Amoebiasis
(Schistosomiasis)

Chronic inflammatory bowel disease
Ulcerative colitis
Crohn's disease

Vascular
Ischaemic colitis

Neoplastic
Benign colonic polyps
Colonic carcinoma
(Lymphomas and other tumours)

Others
Diverticula
(Solitary rectal ulcer)
(Radiation colitis)

Less common conditions are shown in parentheses.

developments in true typhoid and paratyphoid fevers, which more usually present with constitutional symptoms during the bacteraemic phase of the disease.

Salmonellosis is most frequently contracted from infected meats, poultry or milk products, particularly where unhygienic storage or inadequate cooking have been permitted. When an outbreak of the disease occurs it can sometimes be traced to a single infective source, and this may have important implications for the prevention of further dissemination in the community.

SHIGELLA. Patients with bacillary dysentery seen in the United Kingdom have usually contracted the illness when travelling abroad. *Shigella sonnei* is the most frequent organism, and the disease is commonly acquired by ingestion of contaminated food or water. The incubation period is about three days and the patient then develops acute diarrhoea with abdominal discomfort, urgency of defaecation, tenesmus and fever. The motions are initially watery but, in the typical case, soon consist principally of blood and mucus. In severe attacks, dehydration, hypotension, massive intestinal haemorrhage or even perforation may occur. However, most patients recover in a few days with supportive measures only.

Campylobacter jejuni is the commonest pathogen detected by many laboratories

CAMPYLOBACTER JEJUNI. Campylobacters have recently been recognised as an important cause of infectious diarrhoea in man. With the routine use of special culture techniques, campylobacters are isolated from 10-15% of diarrhoeal stools, and are the commonest intestinal pathogen detected by many bacteriological laboratories. The infection may be contracted from live or dead poultry, from domestic pets (particularly puppies), from unpasteurised milk or contaminated water and occasionally from other human cases (particularly between infants). The incubation period of a few days is followed by malaise, headache and fever in many patients, and then by the onset of abdominal pain and diarrhoea, which may be bloody. The illness may be sharp and severe, but usually subsides in under a week; relapse of symptoms is not uncommon. *Campylobacter* enteritis may mimic acute ulcerative colitis quite closely, and bacteriological studies are mandatory to differentiate between these conditions.

Pseudomembranous colitis

The true incidence of this inflammatory disorder of the colon remains unknown, as many cases are mild and self-limited while others are not accurately diagnosed. The condition most commonly develops several days or weeks after the affected patient has received a course of a broad-spectrum antibiotic. Clindamycin and lincomycin have a particularly bad reputation as precipitants of antibiotic-associated pseudomembranous colitis but a wide variety of other agents have been incriminated, including penicillins, cephalosporins, tetracyclines, chloramphenicol and co-trimoxazole. Clinical evidence and experiments in animals suggest that many cases of pseudomembranous colitis are due to overgrowth in the bowel of an enterotoxin-producing strain of *Clostridium difficile.*

The disease tends to affect elderly subjects and typically appears 10 days or so after antibiotic therapy. Fever, abdominal pain and watery diarrhoea, with or without blood, are the usual symptoms. In severe cases the patient may become gravely ill, with abdominal distension, dehydration and hypoproteinaemia. Mild attacks of antibiotic-associated diarrhoea frequently settle after withdrawal of the causative drug.

Amoebiasis

This is a relatively unusual condition in the United Kingdom, but not one to be missed! Like bacillary dysentery, amoebiasis is usually an imported disease, but endemic cases do occur.

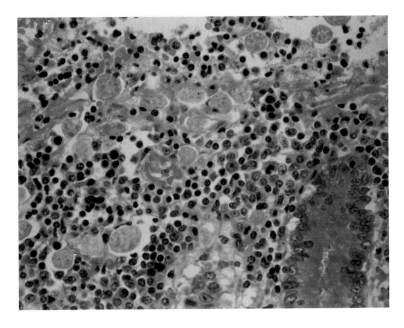

Fig. 15.1 Amoebic dysentery. Parasites may be seen in this rectal biopsy specimen.

The incubation period may be prolonged, and the bowel disturbance can vary from the insidious onset of mild looseness to severe diarrhoea with colonic ulceration and the passage of frank blood and mucus (Fig. 15.1). Systemic disturbance may be minimal in the less severe cases. Occasionally patients develop local complications such as perforation or an inflammatory mass. Hepatic involvement may lead to the development of single or multiple amoebic liver abscesses.

Medical attention may be sought either because of the dysenteric illness or because of symptoms related to hepatic infection; in either event it is likely that special investigations and treatment in hospital will be required.

Chronic inflammatory bowel disease

ULCERATIVE COLITIS. This is the commonest chronic inflammatory bowel disease encountered in the United Kingdom, with a prevalence in the population of roughly one per thousand. The aetiology of ulcerative colitis remains obscure, although many theories have been advanced over the years, including genetic influences, dietary allergy, infection, various immunological disturbances, metabolic dysfunction of the colonic mucosa and even that it could be psychosomatic in origin.

The disease most commonly begins in adolescence or early adult life, though it may start at any age. The inflammatory reaction typically involves the large bowel mucosa (Fig. 15.2), but extension deeper into the gut wall can occur when the attack is severe. The disorder may be confined to the rectum (ulcerative proctitis) or extend upwards in continuity to involve more proximal parts of the colon (Fig. 15.3). The disease proper is always confined to the large bowel, but minor radiological and histological abnormalities may occur in the terminal ileum ('backwash ileitis') when universal colitis is present.

Ulcerative colitis is always confined to the large bowel

A patient in a first attack of ulcerative colitis typically presents with frequent loose stools containing blood and mucus. The severity of bowel disturbance ranges from mild irregularity with minimal bleeding to fulminant bloody diarrhoea with anaemia, electrolyte imbalance and hypovolaemic circulatory collapse. Nocturnal diarrhoea and urgency of defaecation may be particularly troublesome symptoms. Systemic illness is common in moderate or severe cases, and fulminant colitis can rapidly progress to toxic

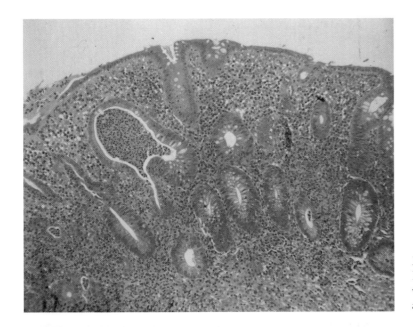

Fig. 15.2 Ulcerative colitis. Note the mucosal inflammation, with loss of surface epithelium and crypt abscess formation.

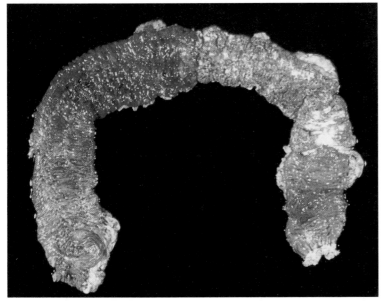

Fig. 15.3 Universal ulcerative colitis.

dilatation or perforation if appropriate treatment is at all delayed.

A minority of patients, perhaps 10% of the total, develop non-colonic manifestations of ulcerative colitis either at the start of their disease or later in its course. These extracolonic features include iritis, skin rashes, seronegative arthritis and various forms of chronic liver disease.

Accurate assessment of ulcerative colitis certainly necessitates out-patient or in-patient hospital investigations. The condition is characterised by remissions and relapses of activity, and so continued hospital supervision is likely to be needed in all but the most trivial of cases. A small minority of patients with chronic ulcerative colitis, particularly those with long-standing universal disease, are at risk of developing colonic carcinoma; this subgroup needs especially careful long-term follow-up if adequate cancer prophylaxis is to be achieved.

CROHN'S DISEASE. This has been discussed in detail in Chapter 13. Crohn's disease is less common than ulcerative colitis, although the true incidence of the condition seems to have been increasing in the United Kingdom until recently. The disease often begins in the second or third decade of life, and the typical clinical features are abdominal pain, loose motions and weight loss. In contrast to ulcerative colitis, any part of the digestive tract may be involved by Crohn's disease, and discontinuous 'skip lesions' are common. The inflammatory reaction is transmural in distribution, and characteristic non-caseating granulomata are present in many cases (Fig. 15.4). More than 50% of patients have some degree of colonic involvement (Fig. 15.5), and in such cases the diarrhoea may contain obvious blood. Complications of the disease are common; these may be local (abscesses, strictures, fistulae) or extra-intestinal (a similar spectrum to the non-colonic manifestations of ulcerative colitis).

> Crohn's disease may involve any part of the digestive tract

Crohn's disease frequently presents in an insidious fashion and diagnosis is often delayed until the patient has been symptomatic for months or even years. With adequate medical and surgical treatment most patients remain in good health for the majority of the time, but problems in management are common and expert long-term supervision is strongly advisable for patients with the disorder.

Ischaemic colitis

This condition is unusual, but sometimes develops in middle-aged and elderly subjects, who often have other evidence of degenerative vascular disease. Clinical features are abdominal pain of sudden onset, followed by diarrhoea containing dark blood and sometimes clots. In severe cases colonic gangrene

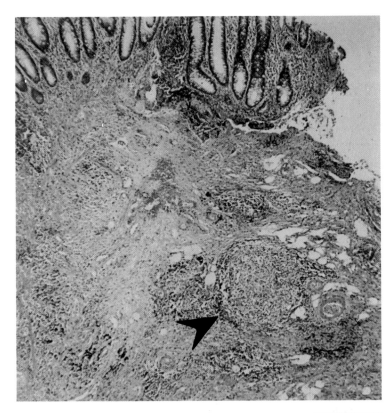

Fig. 15.4 Crohn's disease. Transmural inflammation with granuloma formation (arrowed).

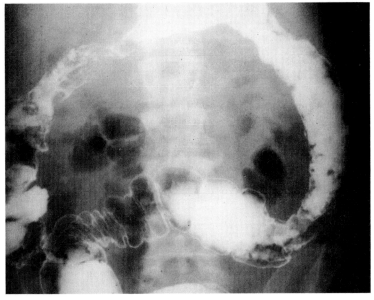

Fig. 15.5 Skip lesions and deep ulceration with abscess formation, due to Crohn's disease, shown on a barium enema.

develops, causing abdominal distension, peritonitis and shock; the mortality is at least 80%. Less severe ischaemia may settle with conservative treatment, but a colonic stricture develops after a few weeks in about half such cases.

Colonic tumours

Benign or malignant tumours of the colon often present with a change in bowel habit and/or rectal bleeding. Bloody diarrhoea may be associated with the presence of large adenomatous polyps or of invasive carcinomas or other malignant growths. When these conditions are suspected, urgent investigation is clearly indicated in order to ensure rapid and effective treatment. Delays in hospital referral and investigation are an important correctable factor in the still high mortality of colonic malignancy. Piles do not cause bloody diarrhoea.

Piles do not cause bloody diarrhoea

Diverticula

Patients with diverticular disease of the colon often have intermittent abdominal pain and loose motions. Bloody diarrhoea can rarely be due to colonic diverticula, but other conditions, particularly tumours, must be carefully excluded before this explanation for the patient's symptoms is accepted. Profuse rectal haemorrhage in elderly subjects is more likely to be coming from vascular anomalies in the colon (angiodysplasia) than from the diverticula which many of these patients also possess.

CLUES FROM THE HISTORY

The following points are worth specific attention when talking to the patient:

PATTERN OF ONSET. Bloody diarrhoea which starts abruptly is likely to be infective in origin, although other conditions such as ulcerative colitis or ischaemic colitis may also begin suddenly.

ASSOCIATED GASTROINTESTINAL DISTURBANCE. Vomiting and abdominal colic point to the likelihood of infection; abdominal pain is a particularly prominent feature of *Campylobacter* enteritis. More persistent bloody diarrhoea with abdominal pain may suggest Crohn's disease of the colon.

CONTACTS, TRIPS ABROAD, NEW FAMILY PETS, UNUSUAL FOODS. All these make a gastrointestinal infection or infestation highly likely.

WEIGHT LOSS. Sudden weight loss may occur in infective enteritis due to anorexia and dehydration, but persistent symptoms and progressive weight loss should suggest inflammatory bowel disease or possibly a disseminated malignancy.

RECENT ABTIBIOTIC TREATMENT. Think of pseudo-membranous colitis, but antibiotics also sometimes exacerbate chronic inflammatory bowel disease.

EXTRA-INTESTINAL FEATURES.. Skin rashes may occur in infective enteritides, but more unusual eruptions, such as erythema nodosum or pyoderma gangrenosum, point to ulcerative colitis or Crohn's disease. Acute arthritis or eye inflammation again suggest the possibility of inflammatory bowel disease.

INSIDIOUS ONSET AND PROGRESSION OF SYMPTOMS. Think of inflammatory bowel disease or a possible tumour; the patient's age and other symptoms may make one of these obviously the more probable.

IRRITABLE BOWEL SYMPTOMS. These may point towards diverticular disease, but keep an open mind as to other possibilities.

HISTORY OF CARDIOVASCULAR DISEASE. Ischaemic bowel disease should be considered if such a patient suddenly develops bloody diarrhoea.

ABNORMALITIES ON EXAMINATION

In many patients with bloody diarrhoea, physical examination will not be particularly helpful in reaching a precise diagnosis. Some features worth especial consideration are:

Fever

This is not a helpful discriminatory physical sign, but suggests either gastrointestinal infection or some other potentially serious inflammatory bowel problem.

Dehydration

Again, this is not a helpful discriminant, but it does indicate that the diarrhoea must be severe enough to induce significant fluid depletion. The physical effects will be exaggerated if vomiting is also present.

Anaemia

The presence of clinically obvious anaemia implies that blood loss has either been profuse or has continued for a considerable period. Patients with ulcerative colitis, Crohn's disease or colonic neoplasms are particularly likely to be anaemic by the time they come to medical attention.

Abdominal findings

Tenderness along the course of the colon is an unhelpful sign, as it may be present in any patient with diarrhoea and bleeding.

Abdominal distension and signs of peritonism clearly indicate an acute and probably serious problem needing special investigation and treatment without delay.

Care should be taken to search for any abdominal mass. If a lump is present in the right iliac fossa, this is likely (in Great Britain at least) to be either a tumour or an inflammatory mass due to Crohn's disease. Masses elsewhere along the course of the large bowel should be thought of as neoplastic until proved otherwise.

Perianal and rectal abnormalities

Always have a look at the anal region. Some perianal abnormality is said to be present in the majority of patients with Crohn's disease of the colon; ulcerated skin tags (Fig. 15.6), fissures and fistulae are particularly common (see Chapter 19).

Rectal examination should be performed if at all possible; it can be omitted only if the patient is in too much discomfort to allow internal examination without an anaesthetic. Every doctor misses an obvious rectal tumour once, but he should feel excessively silly afterwards (and it's bad clinical management!).

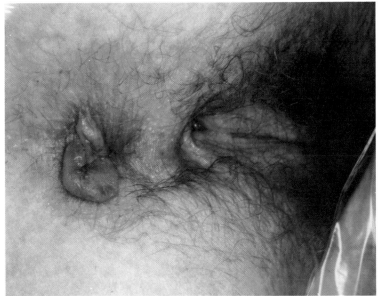

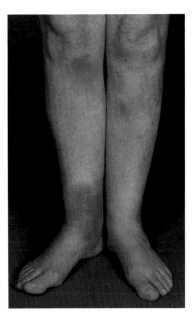

Extra-intestinal abnormalities

These are worth looking for in the context of inflammatory bowel disease. The skin may show typical eruptions such as erythema nodosum (Fig. 15.7) or pyoderma gangrenosum (Fig. 15.8). The common ocular abnormality is acute iritis. Acute non-deforming arthritis of the medium-sized and large joints complicates about 10% of cases of ulcerative colitis or Crohn's disease, and some patients also develop ankylosing spondylitis.

Fig. 15.6 Ulcerated perianal skin tags due to Crohn's disease.

Fig. 15.7 Erythema nodosum on the shins: tender lumps which clear leaving a bruise.

INVESTIGATIONS

In some patients with bloody diarrhoea, simple investigations will suffice to give an accurate diagnosis. The family practitioner will certainly have access to stool culture and routine blood tests, and in some instances may be able to carry out sigmoidoscopy and to order radiological investigations as well. Three criteria should be considered in deciding whether a gastrointestinal specialist's advice is necessary: the patient's physical state, the presumptive diagnosis arrived at from the history and examination, and the results of such tests as can be obtained rapidly from the local laboratory or X-ray department.

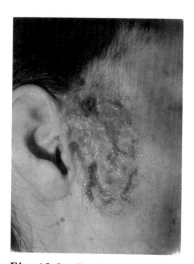

Fig. 15.8 Pyoderma gangrenosum.

A fresh stool specimen from any patient with bloody diarrhoea should be sent for parasites and culture

Stool examination

In any patient with bloody diarrhoea of recent onset, at least three fresh stool specimens should be sent to the microbiology laboratory for parasites and culture.

Microscopy will help to exclude amoebiasis or other parasitic infestation. Bacteriological studies will pick up the common intestinal pathogens within 48 hours. Most laboratories now look for *Campylobacter* species as part of their routine stool examination, but a search for this organism should be specifically requested if it is suspected.

In cases of suspected pseudomembranous colitis, the patient's stool can be tested for *Clostridium difficile* enterotoxin. This is a rather specialised technique involving the use of cell monolayer cultures, but arrangements can usually be made for a sample to be sent away for examination if the test is not available locally. Tell the laboratory that the patient has received a broad-spectrum antibiotic.

Blood tests

Routine blood tests may not be of much diagnostic help in cases of bloody diarrhoea, although occasional diagnostic pointers do emerge. Anaemia or a raised sedimentation rate would indicate a potentially serious illness. A low serum albumin in such patients implies marked exudative protein loss.

Sigmoidoscopy and rectal biopsy

Inspection of the rectum and sigmoid colon with a rigid endoscope is a rapid and valuable diagnostic technique in the assessment of bloody diarrhoea. Any lesions seen can easily be biopsied and the tissue sent for histological examination. The normal rectal mucosa is clear, like the inside of the mouth, with a clear view of the blood vessels in the submucosa. Non-specific mucosal inflammation may be present in an infective colitis, particularly that due to *Campylobacter*. A characteristic lesion is seen in florid pseudomembranous colitis, where the mucosa becomes oedematous and studded with adherent creamy plaques of fibrinous exudate (Fig. 15.9). Sometimes the rectum is not affected, and a negative signoidoscopy does not necessarily exclude the diagnosis.

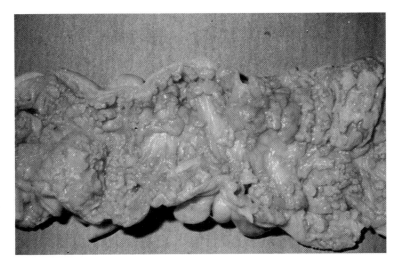

Fig. 15.9   Pseudomembranous colitis.

The typical changes in ulcerative colitis are mucosal erythema and granularity, loss of the normal vascular pattern, contact bleeding and frank ulceration when the disease is severe (Fig. 15.10). In cases where the condition has been present for some time, inflammatory pseudopolyps may be seen (Fig. 15.11).

Crohn's disease of the lower bowel may have a similar appearance, but more often the inflammation is patchy, the rectum may be largely spared, the remaining mucosa adopts a cobblestone appearance (Fig. 15.12), and discrete aphthous or punched-out ulcers may be visible (Fig. 15.13).

If no generalised abnormality is visible with the sigmoidoscope, a careful and systematic search of the lower bowel should be made for a possible neoplasm. The presence of blood coming from higher up the bowel obviously points to some problem in the more proximal colon.

Radiology

A plain abdominal X-ray is usually easily obtainable and sometimes gives useful information in cases of bloody diarrhoea. This is particularly true in patients with inflammatory bowel disease where air in the gut may demonstrate an abnormal mucosal pattern without the need for barium (Fig. 15.14), or where evidence of complications such as toxic dilatation or free perforation may be seen (Fig. 15.15).

Barium studies are very useful when simple infection has been excluded. Active ulcerative colitis (Fig. 15.16) or tumours

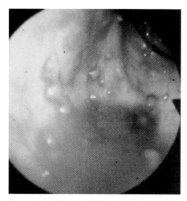

Fig. 15.10   Mild chronic ulcerative colitis, with inflammation, contact bleeding and small pseudopolyps.

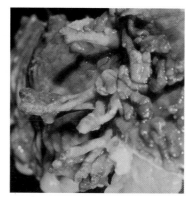

Fig. 15.11   Ulcerative colitis with gross pseudopolyp formation.

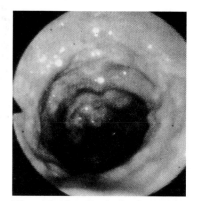

Fig. 15.12   Crohn's disease, with cobblestone mucosa in the transverse colon.

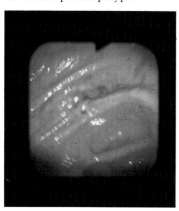

Fig. 15.13   Crohn's disease of the colon with a discrete, punched-out ulcer on a mucosal fold.

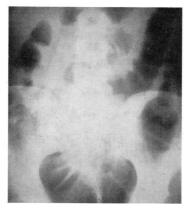

Fig. 15.14   Abnormal mucosal pattern around the splenic flexure, due to Crohn's disease, shown on a plain abdominal X-ray.

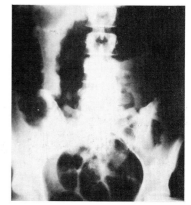

Fig. 15.15   Toxic dilatation of the colon in ulcerative colitis, shown on a plain abdominal X-ray.

(Fig. 15.17) are well demonstrated using the double-contrast technique. If patchy ulceration is seen and skip lesions are present in the colon, the small intestine should be examined for evidence of Crohn's disease (Fig. 15.18).

Colonscopy

After suitable preparation, the whole colon and terminal ileum can be inspected and biopsied using a flexible fibreoptic colonoscope. This is a fairly difficult technique, but is now

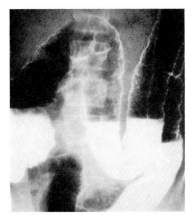

Fig. 15.16 Active universal ulcerative colitis shown on a barium enema.

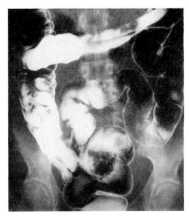

Fig. 15.17 A large polypoid tumour at the rectosigmoid junction, shown on a barium enema.

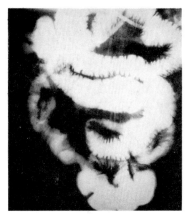

Fig. 15.18 Severe extensive Crohn's disease, with skip lesions and stricture formation, shown on a small bowel intubation enema.

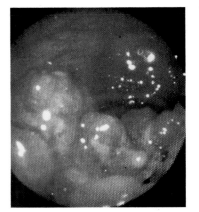

Fig. 15.19 Large adeno-carcinoma in the sigmoid colon, seen at colonoscopy.

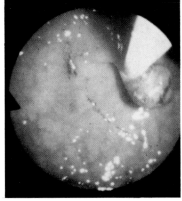

Fig. 15.20 Snare diathermy excision of a benign colonic polyp.

widely practised and should be available in most district general hospitals.

The colonoscope has three important uses: firstly, the whole of the large intestine can be examined by direct vision and proximally situated inflammatory lesions or tumours can be inspected and biopsied (Fig. 15.19). Secondly, colonic polyps may be snared, removed and safely recovered for histological examination with the minimum discomfort and inconvenience to the patient (Fig. 15.20).

MANAGEMENT

Enteric infections and infestations

SALMONELLA INFECTIONS. Most cases of infectious diarrhoea settle after a few days with supportive treatment only. Antibacterial agents are rarely indicated and are reputed to prolong the carrier state in straightforward enteric infections. The treatment of choice in invasive salmonellosis is either co-trimoxazole or ampicillin; patients with a high fever should probably be given a course of either antibiotic.

BACILLARY DYSENTERY. Again antibacterial agents are not usually required as the disease tends to be self-limited. For a severely ill patient, co-trimoxazole in a dose equivalent to two or three tablets twice daily would be appropriate therapy.

CAMPYLOBACTER ENTERITIS. This is usually a short-lived but uncomfortable illness requiring symptomatic management only. Where the patient is severely affected, erythromycin 500 mg twice daily (in adults) will almost invariably check the disease rapidly, quickly clearing the organisms from the stools.

PSEUDOMEMBRANOUS COLITIS. In addition to supportive treatment, the current therapy of choice is vancomycin in a dose of 125-500 mg six-hourly for five to ten days. Metronidazole and ion-exchange resins such as colestipol and cholestyramine have been used, but the clinical response to these agents seems less satisactory.

AMOEBIC DYSENTERY. Metronidazole is the drug of choice in acute amoebic dysentery. It is effective against vegetative parasites in the bowel and the liver, and may be used in a dose of 800 mg thrice daily for 10 days. In chronic infections, where most of the parasites are in the encysted form, diloxanide furoate is more effective.

Inflammatory bowel disease

ULCERATIVE COLITIS. Two principal drugs are used in the therapy of ulcerative colitis: sulphasalazine and corticosteroids. Mildly active disease may settle on treatment with sulphasalazine alone, in a dose of 2-4 g by mouth daily, but the response tends to be rather slow. A more rapid remission is usually obtained if corticosteroids are also used. These may be applied topically to the rectum (as suppositories, foams or retention enemas) in distal disease, or used systemically in a dose equivalent to 20-40 mg of prednisolone daily where the colonic involvement is more extensive. Severly active disease requires hospital admission and careful monitoring of the patient. Intensive therapy with intravenous steroids, together with fluid and electrolyte replacement, parenteral feeding and blood transfusion as necessary, quickly achieves remission of symptoms in the majority of patients, but up to 25% fail to respond and may require urgent colectomy.

If the acute attack does settle with medical treatment, the steroids should be tailed off over a few weeks. Moderate doses of corticosteroid are ineffective in maintaining remission, but sulphasalazine is well established as being helpful in this respect and should be continued as long-term maintenance therapy in the absence of contraindications.

Various other agents have been used in the treatment of ulcerative colitis, and two drugs are particularly worth a mention. Azathioprine is sometimes useful as a steroid-sparing agent in patients who relapse rapidly as glucocorticoids are withdrawn; unfortunately it is not possible to predict in advance which patients are likely to respond to the drug. Disodium cromoglycate was suggested to be helpful in some patients, but critical tests have failed to establish any significant therapeutic role in the majority of patients with ulcerative colitis.

CROHN'S DISEASE. Acute Crohn's disease is treated in much the same way as ulcerative colitis. There is some evidence that, in the active phase, corticosteroids may be the most effective therapy in patients with predominantly small bowel involvement, whereas sulphasalazine may be more helpful in Crohn's disease of the colon.

Once the patient's symptoms have settled, there seems little academic justification to continue with either drug, as neither has been definitely shown to be an effective maintenance treatment. Many patients develop complications such as abscesses or fistulae, and the majority will require surgery at some stage during the course of follow-up. Unfortunately, even extensive resections are not curative and most patients relapse within a few years even when all macroscopic disease has been removed.

Other conditions

ISCHAEMIC COLITIS. Minor episodes of colonic ischaemia may settle with transfusion and supportive therapy, although later

> Sulphasalazine should be continued as long-term maintenance therapy

surgery is sometimes necessary if a tight stricture develops at the site of the vascular lesion. Surgical resection is required when colonic gangrene occurs, but the mortality in such patients is extremely high.

NEOPLASMS. Benign colonic polyps are readily removed by colonoscopic polypectomy. Invasive tumours are usually treated by surgical resection or by-pass unless the disease is extremely advanced.

DIVERTICULA. Bleeding associated with diverticula usually settles spontaneously, although transfusion may be necessary. The associated bowel motility disturbance is subsequently treated along conventional lines with antispasmodics, bulk-forming agents or a high-fibre diet.

FURTHER READING

Anon (1979) Epidemiology: food poisoning and salmonellosis surveillance in England and Wales: 1979. Br Med J 281: 1360-1361.

Kirsner JB, Shorter RG. Recent developments in 'nonspecific' inflammatory bowel disease. N Engl J Med 306: 775-786, 837-848.

Leading Article (1981) Antibiotic-associated colitis: the continuing saga. Br Med J 282: 1913-1914.

Leading Article (1981) Treatment of ulcerative colitis. Br Med J 282: 1255-1256.

Leading Article (1983) Colonoscopy: essential service in a general hospital. Lancet 1: 1311-1312.

Morson BC (1979) Prevention of colorectal cancer. J R Soc Med 72: 83-85.

Symonds J (1983) Campylobacter enteritis in the community. Br Med J 386: 243-244.

Welch CE, Malt RA (1983) Abdominal surgery, part 2. N Engl J Med 308: 685-695.

Willoughby CP, Slack MPE (1982) Campylobacter enteritis. In: Jewell DP (ed) Advanced Medicine, 17. London: Pitman Medical, 128-137.

CHRISTINE LEE

Doctor, I think I'm anaemic

16

Primary disease of the gastrointestinal tract often presents with anaemia. The anaemia may be difficult to detect on clinical examination, but a blood test can provide the first definite evidence of organic disease.

The modern automatic machines which measure haemoglobin also provide a wealth of additional information --look for extra diagnostic clues in the mean corpuscular volume (MCV), the white cell count and the platelet count.

> Automatic machines for measuring haemoglobin produce a wealth of other diagnostic information

DIFFERENTIAL DIAGNOSIS

Blood loss is the commonest cause of anaemia in patients with gastrointestinal disease. To produce anaemia, chronic blood loss must exceed 20 ml per day. The causes of occult gastrointestinal blood loss include carcinoma of the any part of the bowel, peptic ulcer, oesophagitis, inflammatory bowel disease (Crohn's disease or ulcerative colitis), haemorrhoids or infestation with parasites. Brisk haemorrhage provides obvious evidence of the cause of anaemia (Fig. 16.1). Anaemia may also result from poor dietary intake, particularly in alcoholics, the elderly or the strictly vegetarian. Malabsorption of iron, folic acid or vitamin B12 is a less common cause of anaemia, but it may occur in coeliac disease, pernicious anaemia, ulcerative colitis, Crohn's disease, bacterial overgrowth of the small bowel, lymphoma or intestinal tuberculosis. Chronic liver disease may cause portal hypertension with anaemia due to hypersplenism. Finally, virtually any systemic illness may cause a non-specific anaemia -- the anaemia of chronic disease.

Table 16.1 Causes of anaemia and gastrointestinal disease

Blood loss
Inadequate diet
Malabsorption
Liver disease
Chronic illness

CLUES FROM THE HISTORY

Mild anaemia may be asymptomatic, but as the haemoglobin drops so the patient develops progressive exhaustion, with breathlessness and even high-output heart failure.

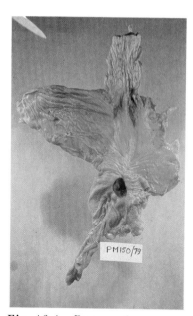

Fig. 16.1 Post mortem stomach and oesophagus. The patient was thought to be dying from bleeding varices, but the gastric ulcer was the real problem.

Not all Indians are vegans: obtain a dietary history to exclude other causes of anaemia

Iron deficiency alone can cause unusual symptoms: pruritus or pica. The latter may result in bizarre dietary supplements or fancies, for example coal, ice or pickles.

In a male, or postmenopausal female, iron deficiency anaemia is usually due to gastrointestinal blood loss. Thus the doctor should ask such patients positively about alteration in bowel habit, whether there is blood in the stool either as melaena (like tar) or as fresh blood in the pan, or whether the patient has noticed piles. Symptoms of indigestion or abdominal pain may be related to a malignant gastric ulcer, carcinoma of the pancreas, a peptic ulcer or oesophagitis.

In a menstruating woman menorrhagia must be considered before gastrointestinal causes are sought. However, it is difficult to quantify menstrual blood loss, so enquiries concerning gastrointestinal symptoms should always be made.

A dietary history is particularly helpful if an alcoholic or an elderly person presents with folate deficiency. Although an inadequate intake of meat and fresh fruit and vegetables can cause profound anaemia, it is dangerous to diagnose a dietary deficiency of iron.

Malabsorption may present as a profound wasting illness with loss of weight and greasy stools due to steatorrhoea. However, in the adult it often presents with anaemia. A patient with coeliac disease may give a history of always being smaller than the peer group and being known as 'titch' at school. Pernicious anaemia is frequently associated with a sore tongue and minor neurological symptoms such as paraesthesiae; there is commonly a family history. A partial gastrectomy is often followed, years later, by either iron or vitamin B12 deficiency.

Strict vegetarians, particularly Hindu vegans, may have a dietary vitamin B12 deficiency; not all Indians are vegans and it is important to obtain a careful dietary history because of the other causes of anaemia 'special' to this group -- parasite infestation, abdominal tuberculosis and thalassaemia.

A history of excessive alcohol intake may raise the possibility of not only folate deficiency but also of hypersplenism. Progressive ill health and weight loss may suggest a chronic illness, for example advanced malignancy, with anaemia due to chronic disease.

ABNORMALITIES ON EXAMINATION

General observations about the patient may give vital clues. If the patient is Indian, particularly female, this puts a dietary cause high on the list. A small, underweight patient might suggest coeliac disease. The colour of the skin can have a yellow tint in pernicious anaemia and the association of blue eyes and premature greying hair is common. The tongue mucosa is flattened, with associated angular stomatitis, in iron deficiency (Fig. 16.2), and in vitamin B12 and folate deficiency there may be an angry glossitis with fissuring. Nails may show breakages in iron deficiency, but koilonychia (Fig. 16.3) is found only in a patient with prolonged iron deficiency.

In the cardiovascular system signs of severe anaemia may show as an ejection systolic murmur with later congestive

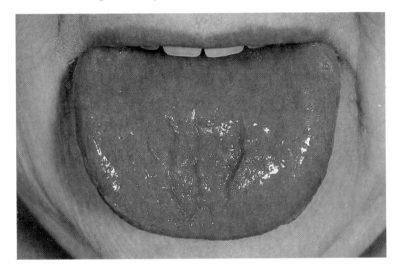

Fig. 16.2 A smooth tongue and angular stomatitis in a woman with chronic iron deficiency.

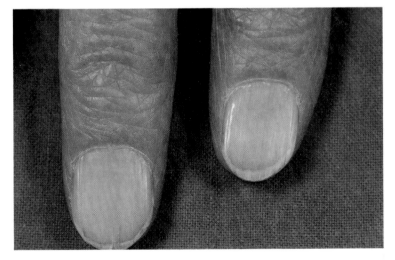

Fig. 16.3 Koilonychia.

	TEST	NORMALS COULTER COUNTER MALE	FEMALE
6·1	WBC X 10⁹/l	4.0-11	4.0-11
5·47	RBC X10¹²/l	4.5-6.5	3.8-5.8
10·1	Hgb g/dl	13.5-17.5	11.5-15.5
·354	Hct l/l	0.4-0.54	0.37-0.47
64·	MCV fl	80.95	80.95
18·5	MCH pg	27-32	27-32
28·8	MCHC g/dl	31-35	31-35

Fig. 16.4 Iron deficiency anaemia: note the low MCV.

	TEST	NORMALS COULTER COUNTER MALE	FEMALE
4·01	WBC X 10⁹/l	4.0-11	4.0-11
4·11	RBC X10¹²/l	4.5-6.5	3.8-5.8
8·6	Hgb g/dl	13.5-17.5	11.5-15.5
·351	Hct l/l	0.4-0.54	0.37-0.47
114·	MCV fl	80.95	80.95
17·9	MCH pg	27-32	27-32
29·1	MCHC g/dl	31-35	31-35

Fig. 16.5 Macrocytic anaemia: note the raised MCV.

Elevated white cell count suggests a primary haematological problem or a reactive change due to inflammation or infection

Macrocytosis may suggest unsuspected alcoholism

cardiac failure, ankle oedema, raised jugular venous pressure and crepitations at lung bases. Tenderness in the epigastrium may occur in association with peptic ulcer, but it is not a specific sign. Malignancy may be detected as irregular hepatosplenomegaly or as a palpable abdominal mass. Rectal examination can be helpful; it may reveal piles, a rectal mass or melaena.

An examination of the central nervous system could be helpful if pernicious anaemia is suspected. Subacute combined degeneration of the cord may impair position sense, so that the patient cannot keep balance when standing with heels together and eyes closed.

INVESTIGATIONS

The full blood count, blood film and ESR provide crucial information. The level of anaemia will be quantified. The mean cell volume (MCV), together with film appearance, will indicate if the anaemia is hypochromic and microcytic, or macrocytic. The normal MCV is 76-96 fl, but there is a small variation between laboratories. Values less than 76 fl suggest iron deficiency (Fig. 16.4), whereas values greater than 96 fl indicate macrocytosis (Fig 16.5). Anaemia with a normal MCV indicates either a mixed deficiency or the anaemia of chronic disease. An elevated platelet count usually indicates active bleeding or malignancy. An elevated white cell count suggests either a primary haematological problem or a reactive change due to inflammation or infection.

If iron deficiency is suspected, the serum iron and total iron binding capacity should be measured and stools should be examined for occult blood (Fig. 16.6). If blood loss is suspected or confirmed, further examinations of the gastrointestinal tract are necessary: for example barium meal, barium enema, upper gastrointestinal endoscopy or sigmoidoscopy. It is at this stage that the patient should be referred to the gastroenterologist (Fig. 16.7).

Macrocytosis, often in the absence of anaemia, may indicate unsuspected excessive alcohol intake. Together with the enzyme gamma-glutamyl transpeptidase, macrocytosis is a sensitive, but non-specific, screen for alcoholism.

Macrocytosis in the presence of anaemia is usually caused by folate or vitamin B12 deficiency. The blood count often shows an associated leucopenia and thrombocytopenia; the blood film

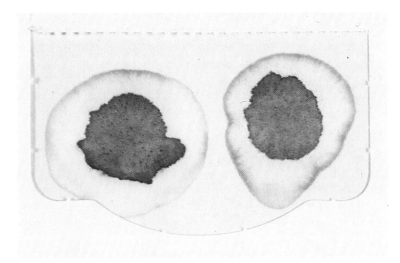

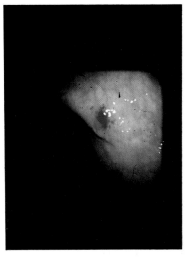

Fig. 16.6   The Haemoccult slide detects occult bleeding by the blue colour, a system that can be performed in the surgery.

Fig. 16.7   Angiodysplasia of the colon: a leash of submucosal blood vessels that can cause chronic occult bleeding in the elderly.

shows oval macrocytes with hypersegmentation of polymorphs. Vitamin B12 and folate levels should be measured. Both the serum and red cell folate should be measured, as the latter is a more accurate reflection of body stores. Where there is associated neurological change or thrombocytopenia it is important to start treatment early. A bone marrow examination should be performed immediately, and if this shows megaloblastic change both vitamin B12 and folic acid should be given before the results of assay levels are available. If this non-invasive investigation demonstrates malabsorption the patient can be referred to a gastroenterologist for further investigation of the small intestine.

If a megaloblastic anaemia is secondary to folate deficiency a small intestinal biopsy is usually required. The jejunal mucosa is abnormal and flattened in coeliac disease.

Vitamin B12 and iron deficiency often occur many years after gastrectomy or partial gastrectomy. Iron deficiency may be due to a number of problems: non-repletion of iron stores after peptic ulceration or the surgical procedure; stomal ulceration; surgical diversion of food away from the proximal small intestine where iron is absorbed; inadequate gastric acid to convert Fe^{3+} to Fe^{2+}; or poor nutrition due to anorexia after gastric surgery (Fig. 16.8). Malabsorption of vitamin B12 after gastric surgery is secondary either to reduced intrinsic factor secretion by the gastric remnant or to bacterial overgrowth of

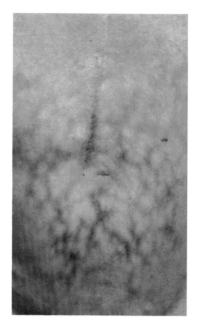

Fig. 16.8 Erythema ab igne. The patient had chronic abdominal pain due to stomal ulcer after unsuccessful gastric surgery for a duodenal ulcer. He also had anaemia due to iron deficiency.

the small intestine due to a surgical blind loop. The blood film appearances may be confusing in these patients, often with a normal mean cell volume; the levels of iron, total iron binding capacity and vitamin B12 have to be measured.

The ß thalassaemia trait causes a microcytic anaemia which can be confused with iron deficiency. ß thalassaemia is relatively common in people who come from anywhere between the Mediterranean and the Indian subcontinent. In such patients, any iron deficiency should be excluded by iron and total iron binding capacity examination, or examination of the bone marrow for iron stores. The iron deficiency should be treated before a diagnostic haemoglobin electrophoresis is performed. This is important because, in the presence of iron deficiency, the electrophoresis may give a false-negative result.

MANAGEMENT

Iron deficiency should be treated not only to raise the haemoglobin to normal levels but also to restore body iron stores. Treatment can be started while the casue of the iron deficiency is being investigated -- the diagnosis of occult gastrointestinal haemorrhage is often a long process! Ferrous sulphate 200 mgs tds should be given for three months after the haemoglobin has returned to normal, to ensure that the stores are replete.

Folate deficiency should be treated with folic acid 5 mg daily. Where the cause is a dietary deficiency a three-month course is adequate, provided dietary education is successful. However, in malabsorption folic acid should be given until the underlying cause has responded to treatment. This pharmacological dose of folic acid will mask the haematological signs of vitamin B12 deficiency, but the neurological damage will continue. There is no place for a trial of folic acid therapy without prior measurement of the serum concentration of both vitamin B12 and folic acid.

Pernicious anaemia should be treated for life with vitamin B12 injections. Initially, vitamin B12 should be given to restore body iron stores (for example 1000 μg hydroxycobalamin, five intramuscular injections over a two-week period). Thereafter an injection should be given every three months for the rest of the patient's life. Where there is a dietary cause of vitamin B12 deficiency, as in vegans, vitamin B12 can be given by mouth as cyanocobalamin (Cytacon). One tablet (50 μg) weekly with

There is no place for a trial of folic acid therapy

Pernicious anaemia should be treated for life with vitamin B12 injections

Sunday lunch is adequate and it is probably advisable for the whole family to take the vitamin on a regular basis if the houshold maintains a strict vegetarian diet.

In Crohn's disease it is often necessary to keep the patient on maintenance vitamin B12, iron and folic acid.

There may be a secondary anaemia in association with gastrointestinal disease. This is an anaemia which is characterised by a low serum iron and a low total iron binding capacity; when the bone marrow is examined iron is present in reticuloendothelial cells but cannot be used by developing red cells. This is known as 'iron-block' anaemia or the anaemia of chronic disease. Such anaemias will not respond to iron; it is treatment and reversal of the underlying cause which results in a normal haemoglobin. Treatment with iron is useless for these patients.

FURTHER READING

Baker SJ, DeMaeyer EM (1979) Nutritional anemia: its understanding and control with special reference to the work of the World Health Organization. Am J Clin Nutr 32: 368-417.

Finch CA, Huebers H (1982) Perspectives in iron metabolism. N Engl J Med 306: 1520-1528.

Hardcastle JD, Farrands PA, Balfour TW, Chamberlain J, Amar SS, Sheldon MG (1983) Controlled trial of faecal occult blood testing in the detection of colorectal cancer. Lancet 2: 1-4.

Leader (1980) Preventing iron deficiency. Lancet i: 1117-1118.

Leicester RJ, Lightfoot A, Millar J, Colin-Jones DG, Hunt RH (1983) Accuracy and value of the Hemoccult test in symptomatic patients. Br Med J 286: 673-674.

Doctor, I suffer from terrible wind

Healthy human beings pass approximately 0.5 litre of gas through their gut each day, though there is an extremely wide individual variation. The major source of intestinal gas is swallowed air, which may be either belched upwards or passed through the intestine, emerging as flatus. Oxygen is rapidly absorbed. The major component of swallowed air passed as flatus is nitrogen. The two other important sources of intestinal gas are the interaction of bicarbonate and acid in the stomach, which generates carbon dioxide (CO_2), and bacterial fermentation, which generally occurs in the large bowel and produces hydrogen, CO_2 and methane.

The study of intestinal gas in the past has been rather imprecise, but it is now known that there is only about 200 ml of gas in the gastrointestinal tract at any one time. It is possible to measure the different components of intestinal gas, either directly in flatus or indirectly. Hydrogen can readily be measured in exhaled air and it provides some indicator of intestinal bacterial activity; breath methane can also be measured but is very variable.

Overall there is no qualitative or quantitative difference between the intestinal gas of patients complaining of wind and that of healthy individuals, and most of the symptoms which people report are probably the result of motility disorders. Patients whose principal complaint is wind are often not suffering from any serious disorder and reassurance may be all that is necessary to resolve symptoms completely. It is very important to avoid using potent drugs, which may worsen symptoms or make evaluation of diagnostic tests difficult, before a patient has been fully assessed (Table 17.1). On the other hand, it may be necessary to offer patients some treatment while awaiting developments or the results of clinical tests (Table 17.2). Generally speaking the use of antacids,

Most of the symptoms of wind result from motility disorders

Table 17.1   Drugs to avoid before a definite diagnosis

Drugs which heal peptic disease
H$_2$-receptor antagonists:
  ranitidine
  cimetidine
Liquorice derivatives:
  carbenoxolone
  deglycyrrhizinised liquorice
Tricyclic antidepressants:
  amitriptyline
  imipramine
  trimipramine
Other agents:
  colloidal bismuth
  sucralfate
  alginates

Atropinic agents
Propantheline
Hyoscine
Dicyclomine
Pirenzepine

Bile acids
Ursodeoxycholic acid
Chenodeoxycholic acid

Other agents
Oxethazaine
Sodium bicarbonate
Milk
Calcium antacids

antispasmodics, dimethicone, bulking agents or tranquillisers should not interfere with the correct diagnosis and management of patients.

Patients who complain of wind as their major problem generally fall into one of three categories:

1. Excess belching and abdominal bloating (Table 17.3).
2. Abdominal bloating and excess flatus.
3. Foul belching.

A full relevant history may well reveal other problems which require investigation in their own right, such as weight loss, jaundice, rectal bleeding or symptomatic steatorrhoea. A drug history is important as agents such as antibacterials are common causes of gastrointestinal upset. A full alcohol and social history often reveals the trigger for symptoms, and cigarette smokers are known to have more gastrointestinal complaints than non-smokers.

General physical and abdominal examination should be performed but are usually unhelpful; digital examination of the rectum and proctosigmoidoscopy are best reserved for those patients where there is some further specific indication.

Supplementary investigation may be required, but there is no global recommendation which can be made. Each patient requires individual assessment. Full blood count with indices, 'liver function' tests including gamma glutamyl trans-peptidase, serum thyroxine, upper digestive endoscopy, barium swallow, barium meal, small bowel meal, barium enema, oral cholecystogram or gallbladder ultrasound may all be useful in individual patients.

However, clinical tests are often performed primarily to reassure that there is no serious problem. It is important to avoid over-investigation as this may itself both generate further symptoms and lead to the inappropriate detection of silent abnormalities. It is thought that about half of our elderly population have either diverticular disease or gallstones or both.

BELCHING AND BLOATING

Aerophagia

Every swallow will take a few millilitres of air into the stomach. If people swallow excessively, then it follows that excessive quantities of air are available to be belched back. Humans are rather badly designed in that a frequent response to belching is to swallow more air, so that a vicious cycle can be set up. This is much the commonest cause of belching and patients can sometimes give an impressive display of the physiological mechanism during consultation, as they try to impress the physician with the severity of their disorder. Explanation and reassurance should be effective, though some patients are extraordinarily resistant to accepting the harmless nature of their problem. Excessive air swallowing can be a feature of anxiety state and this is frequently obvious from the general demeanour of the patient. Explanation and treatment with a minor tranquilliser, such as diazepam, is usually effective. Alternatively, a peppermint will relax the gastro-oesophageal sphincter, which may allow controlled release of gas from the stomach. This relief of epigastric distension may stop further air-swallowing. This mechanism may explain the commercial success of after-dinner mints!

Drug induced symptoms

Almost any drug therapy may cause gastrointestinal disturbance. Antibiotic therapy is particularly notorious for doing this. Symptoms usually resolve when the offending drug is discontinued or substituted. Sometimes fungal overgrowth may occur, which can be diagnosed by inspection of the mouth for thrush or by oesophagoscopy. Topical treatment with oral nystatin or amphotericin B is generally successful, but ketoconazole is a useful new addition to the antifungal armamentarium. Digoxin, sulphasalazine and cholestyramine are all agents well known for their propensity to cause gastric intolerance. There are few agents which can be completely exonerated from blame. It is worth while remembering that the patient may be taking drugs different from those recently prescribed.

Gastric surgery

A past history of gastric surgery may be relevant. After peptic ulcer surgery patients may develop recurrent ulceration, which is best diagnosed by endoscopy. In addition, the reduction of gastric acid output and the possible construction of blind loops predisposes to bacterial overgrowth and fermentation. Operations for hiatus hernia and reflux oesophagitis may

Table 17.2 Drugs for wind

Antacids
Magnesium trisilicate mixture
Aluminium hydroxide gel
Magnesium plus aluminium
 mixtures

Dimethicone (a deflatulent)

Antispasmodics
Mebeverine
Dicyclomine
Metoclopramide

Tranquillisers
Diazepam
Lorazepam
Chlorpromazine

Table 17.3 Causes of belching and bloating

Aerophagia
Anxiety state
Drug side effects
Diet, e.g. alcohol, lactose
 intolerance
Sporadic foods, e.g. cucumbers
Non-specific dyspepsia
Peptic ulcers
Oesophagitis
Gastritis
Duodenitis
Ascites
Pregnancy
Coeliac disease
Gastric surgery
Rolling hiatus hernia
Pernicious anaemia
Myocardial infarction

construct a tight gastro-oesophageal junction which does not permit normal belching; this problem is difficult to manage but such patients may respond to deflatulent agents, such as an antacid containing dimethicone.

Lactose intolerance

Lactose intolerance is caused by deficiency of intestinal lactase. It is a common cause of digestive complaints in patients from Mediterranean, eastern and tropical countries, but not in those from northern Europe. Lactose intolerance is relevant only when it accompanies other gut diseases, such as ulcerative colitis. If it is suspected, a simple test is to persuade the patient to drink at least a pint of milk, stand back and see if symptoms are reproduced over the ensuing few hours. Complete exclusion of lactose from the diet requires quite a considerable manipulation, because milk is included in various prepared products. Symptomatic relief encourages compliance with a milk-free regimen.

> Lactose intolerance is relevant only when it accompanies other gut diseases, such as ulcerative colitis

Alcohol

No doctor may need feel apologetic about suspecting alcohol as a cause for a wide variety of digestive and other symptoms. If the history or physical examination suggest this is likely to be a problem, investigations likely to be helpful include serum alcohol, gamma glutamyl transpeptidase and mean corpuscular volume, all of which tend to be elevated in alcoholism. The known association between alcohol and both peptic ulcer and portal hypertension makes endoscopy a prudent further investigation. For patients presenting to the doctor with physical complaints related to alcohol consumption the most important aspect of health care is to persuade them to stop, or at least reduce, drinking. This is much more effective than a programme of investigation for the multitude of complaints that they tend to produce.

Peptic ulceration

Some patients with wind will have active peptic disease such as duodenal and gastric ulcers, oesophagitis, gastritis or duodenitis. If there is a high index of suspicion for these conditions, investigation with endoscopy or a barium meal will be necessary. It is essential that ulcer-healing treatments are not commenced before such investigation, if the results are to be interpretable.

Other diseases

Patients with a rolling hiatus hernia (Fig. 17.1) can give a very characteristic story of progressive abdominal bloating suddenly relieved by belching a large quantity of air. This probably results from release of gaseous distension in the partially obstructed gastric fundus. Carcinoma of the stomach or colon may occasionally present initially as very benign and non-

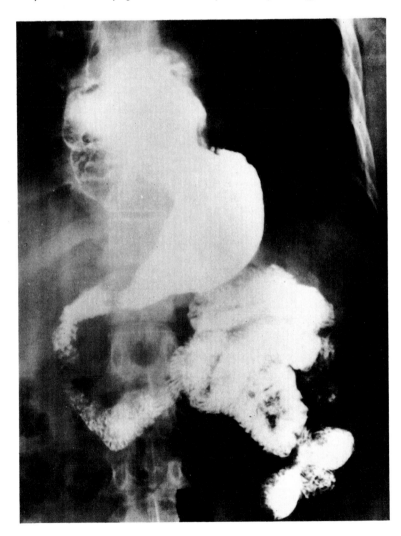

Fig. 17.1 A rolling hiatus hernia with the fundus of the stomach incarcerated above the diaphragm, shown on a barium meal.

Do not investigate the
gallbladder unless there are
definite symptoms: biliary colic,
pancreatitis, a history of
jaundice or previous biliary
surgery

specific complaints. The relationship between flatulent
dyspepsia and gallstones is problematical. It is much better not
to perform investigation of the gallbladder unless there are
accompanying definite symptoms such as biliary colic,
pancreatitis, a history of jaundice or previous biliary surgery.

Though both patient and doctor may be convinced that
symptoms originate from the gastrointestinal tract this may not
be the case. Myocardial infarction is the most embarrassing
missed diagnosis. It should also be remembered that about a
third of patients with pernicious anaemia have vague digestive
complaints which are abolished as soon as vitamin B12
injections are given.

FOUL BELCHING

Patients may complain bitterly about the bad taste of their
eructation. It is always worth while looking for dental caries:
not only do rotting teeth smell bad but their owner will be
unable to chew properly, which can itself cause problems.

Bacterial decay can generate malodorous gases. This can
occur in oesophageal retention, seen with stricture or achalasia;
in gastric outflow obstruction, which can cause retention of a
pool of decaying gastric contents; when carcinoma of the
stomach causes a gastrocolic fistula (Fig. 17.2); and with
bacterial overgrowth of the upper bowel. If these problems are
suspected then barium studies, endoscopy and aspiration and
culture of the appropriate area may all be required.
Mechanical problems will probably require surgical correction,
but short-term relief of symptoms can be obtained by a short
course of oxytetracycline or metronidazole by mouth.

Hepatic or renal failure cause
characteristic foetor

Finally, constipation may cause dyspepsia and foetor,
resulting in foul belching. Hepatic failure or renal failure also
cause a characteristic and unpleasant foetor, which may also be
associated with dyspepsia.

BLOATING AND EXCESS FLATUS

Common causes of this problem include aerophagia and
various dietary components including alcohol and lactose.
Certain foods are notorious for causing excess flatus; beans
certainly do so, as does any increase in dietary fibre. Some
patients are unable to tolerate a high-fibre diet because of the

increased colonic gas production, which is due to normal bacterial degradation of the fibre within the colon. Paradoxically a low-fibre diet and the ensuing constipation may also lead to a complaint of abdominal discomfort and excess flatus. Explanation, reassurance and dietary manipulation are all that are required for the majority of patients.

Irritable bowel syndrome

Various motility disturbances are grouped together under this heading. They are generally considered to arise from the small bowel and colon. The patient is characteristically a young adult or middle-aged; women seem to be affected more than men. A characteristic history is of abdominal discomfort, with the frequent passage of loose stools accompanied by excess flatus and mucus in the morning. The bowel habit is often undisturbed during the rest of the day. Patients may describe

Some patients with irritable bowel syndrome caused by a high-fibre diet cannot tolerate the increased output of flatus per rectum

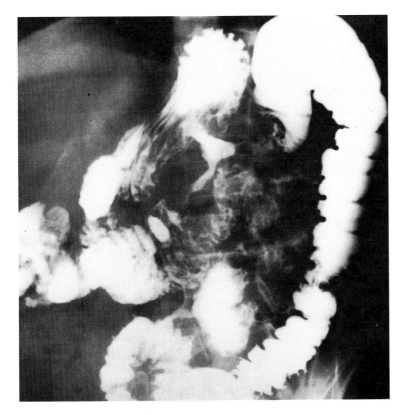

Fig. 17.2 Carcinoma of the stomach causing gastrocolic fistula, which allows faecal contamination of the stomach.

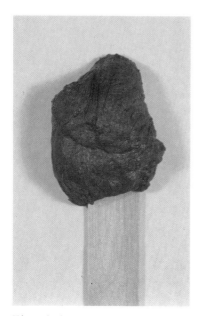

Fig. 17.3 A greasy stool of steatorrhoea.

A floating stool does not automatically mean steatorrhoea

Major causes of steatorrhoea are gastric surgery, coeliac disease and pancreatic insufficiency

colic relieved by bowel action. Weight loss is unusual. Rectal bleeding may be reported because of associated anal fissures or haemorrhoids, but it should never be dismissed without investigation.

Often these patients can be recognised by their characteristic clinical presentation: they are frequently tense and anxious. How far to pursue examination and investigation is always a problem as investigation is a potent cause for reinforcement of symptoms in some patients (see Chapter 6). Although in many of these patients the pain responds to a high-fibre diet, some continue to complain as they cannot tolerate the increased output of flatus per rectum.

Steatorrhoea

Normally fat is absorbed entirely in the jejunum and less than 18 mmol per day is excreted in the stool from dietary and endogenous sources. If fat is not digested and absorbed, it will be fermented by intestinal bacteria with the production of hydrogen, methane and CO_2, together with irritant volatile fatty acids which cause diarrhoea. The result of this sequence of events is clinical steatorrhoea, with the patient complaining of weight loss and frequent, pale, offensive and bulky stools which are difficult to flush away (Fig. 17.3).

Exhaustive American research has shown that floating of stools on water is not due to fat, but to gas trapped in the stool itself. A floating stool does not automatically mean steatorrhoea, although most fatty stools do float, as they also contain gas!

Although many ingenious investigations have been invented to avoid the problem of stool collections, this remains the only accurate way of quantifying steatorrhoea. Steatorrhoea is defined as a faecal fatty acid secretion exceeding 7 g (18 mmol) per day whilst the subject is eating a normal diet containing 70-100 g of fat per day. The three major causes of steatorrhoea are gastric surgery, coeliac disease and pancreatic insufficiency: profound steatorrhoea is generally due to pancreatic disease.

CONCLUSION

Patients will complain of wind when they are suffering from a wide variety of different symptoms whose exact nature needs to be determined before any rational policy of management can be constructed. Intestinal gas itself probably has little significance for the vast majority of these patients and it can be very successfully managed by explanation and the judicious use of the drugs listed in Table 17.2. In these patients, sins of commission are much more frequent than sins of omission. Inappropriate treatment may either make a full diagnosis impossible or cause more problems.

Intestinal gas itself has little significance for the majority of patients

FURTHER READING

Bouchier IAD (1982) Gastroenterology, 3rd ed. London: Baillière Tindall.

Horrocks JC, De Dombal FT (1978) Clinical presentation of patients with 'dyspepsia'. Gut 19: 19-26.

Levitt MD (1980) Intestinal gas production: recent advances in flatology. N Engl J Med 302: 1474-1475.

Levitt MD, Bonn JH (1978) Intestinal gas. In: Sleisinger MH, Fordtran JS (eds) Gastrointestinal Disease, pp 387-92. Philadelphia: WB Saunders.

Shuster M (1981) Gastrointestinal motility disorders. Med Clin N Am 65: 1109-1145.

Spring JA, Buss DH (1977) Three centuries of alcohol in the British diet. Nature 270: 567-572

JOHN BULL

18

Doctor, I'm constipated

One of the great 'British diseases' is an obsession with the bowels, with an associated addiction to 'something to open the bowels'. Many of these patients will have no serious problem other than the unfulfilled expectation of a daily bowel action.

DIFFERENTIAL DIAGNOSIS

Classification of any condition is only useful if it makes remembering its causes easier. Classifictions of the causes of constipation are numerous and arbitrary, but they are summarised in Table 18.1.

The differential diagnosis includes the potentially fatal (large bowel carcinoma), the banal ('simple constipation') and the 'bizarre' (cathartic colon).

Most commonly the patient will have one of the so-called functional disorders (which probably all amount to the same disease, whose origin is in the low-fibre diet of Western man): the irritable or 'irritated' bowel syndrome, which is frequently associated with a depressive illness. The depressed patient often presents with gastrointestinal complaints, frequently including constipation.

Drugs and spontaneous metabolic disturbances are a potent cause of constipation. Of the metabolic causes, bear in mind hypokalaemia (especially from the potent potassium-losing diuretics) and hypercalcaemia, but above all myxoedema.

The bowel habits of the population are many and varied: the normal range of bowel actions (appropriately assessed in the large workforce of a sausage factory in west London) is from three actions a week to three actions a day. Some people are happy with their lot, others are concerned that their habit is 'abnormal'. When the latter group present we call the condition 'simple' constipation. If this diagnosis is correct (that is, there is no other cause), perhaps we should be asking the question 'Why is this patient presenting now?'.

Depressed patients often present with gastrointestinal symptoms, including constipation

CLUES FROM THE HISTORY

The patient's basic details are an important source of clues: age, sex and occupation. An older man of 75 years presenting with constipation will make us think of carcinoma, whereas in a 21-year-old girl the problem is much more likely to be that she is on a slimming diet; a young man of 25 may just have started a sedentary job; an immigrant may have recently arrived in this country and changed his diet. I have seen a number of patients who have suddenly changed from yam, cassava and beans to fish and chips -- a sure recipe for disaster.

Always ask about past history. Unless you ask, a patient may not divulge that constipation is a recurrent problem; he will not tell you about previous illnesses and operations, especially if he considers them irrelevant.

After a preliminary canter into the basic details, the most important thing is to discover exactly what is worrying the patient. Is this a new problem, or has it just come on? If the latter, does the patient ascribe it to anything in particular? The patient is often wrong, but needs to blame something and may give you a clue. A description of the stool as 'hard', 'soft', 'rabbit droppings', 'toothpaste' may sometimes be given by the patient, or you may be able to offer these descriptions as a guide. It is sometimes helpful to see a specimen: it may be the only way to know what is going on. 'Rabbit droppings' and 'toothpaste' are frequently the stools of the irritable bowel syndrome sufferer, but they are not diagnostic - only a clue.

Particularly in constipation of recent onset, one must look for other symptoms, especially rectal bleeding, passage of mucus, tenesmus, weight loss or pain. Anal pain is most commonly due to the presence of a fissure (not piles), and this may well induce constipation. Abdominal pain is usually of less help. Any sort of constipation may cause aching pain, often relieved by defaecation. Colicky pain, however, may indicate an obstructive lesion, but the lack of it does not exclude obstruction.

The next hurdle in the history is the patient's drug cupboard. The drugs you think the patient is taking are easy, but he may not actually be consuming them. It is the other medicaments which are often elusive. What about 'Uncle Harry's DF118, that I always take for my back', or 'Senokot, I've taken that for years'.

It is also useful to delve briefly into the diet. When asked what they eat, patients frequently give you a rundown of what

Table 18.1 Differential diagnosis of constipation

Low-roughage diet
Constitutionally 'lazy' bowel
Slimming diet
Spastic colon
Irritable bowel
Diverticular disease of the colon

Painful anal lesion

Persistently ignoring 'call to stool'

Immobility

Depression

Metabolic
Myxoedema
Low potassium
High calcium

Drugs
Narcotic analgesics
Aluminium-containing antacids
Tricyclic antidepressants
Purgative abuse

Colonic obstruction
Cancer

Hirschprung's disease presenting in the adult

they have had for breakfast, lunch and tea. An exhaustive dietary history is usually a waste of time and it is best to ask a few direct questions about wholemeal bread, breakfast cereals, vegetables and fruit, in order to assess the dietary fibre intake.

Next we must look for clues to some of the conditions which cause secondary constipation. As I mentioned before, depression is common, but in many patients it is not obvious and clues have to be actively sought. Can we detect a history of early morning waking, diurnal mood swings, episodes of weeping or verging on it (this is seldom volunteered spontaneously by a patient presenting with constipation!), dry mouth or decrease in libido? Myxoedema is a well-worn catch and, especially if the cause is not obvious, it is worth asking about weight gain, tolerance of cold and alteration in skin or hair texture. Even a thyroidectomy or treatment with radioactive iodine can be forgotten.

ABNORMALITIES ON EXAMINATION

The last two conditions mentioned in the history may be the first encountered on examination. Depression and myxoedema may be 'diagnosed' on the initial impression of the patient as he walks into the room, from the flatness of affect or the myxoedema facies (Fig. 18.1).

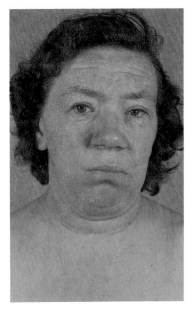

Fig. 18.1 The facial appearance in myxoedema.

Formal examination should include general examination, looking for any clues that may offer themselves, in particular pallor which may be due to anaemia, a sinister complication in any patient presenting with constipation.

Inspection of the abdomen is not usually a great help, although malignant disease may be suspected from obvious masses, wasting or ascites. On palpation malignant masses may be felt either in the bowel or as secondary deposits in the liver. Malignant disease, however, is not the commonest cause of a palpable abdominal mass: in most patients with constipation the caecum and/or the sigmoid colon is palpable, the first filled with faeces and the second in spasm. Sometimes a so-called 'diverticular mass' can be felt and may easily be confused with a malignant mass. A noteworthy sign in the irritable bowel syndrome is the 'squelchy' caecum; again, this is not diagnostic, but it is a clue.

Rectal examination is a must. It will usually reveal the consistency of the faeces. The normal habit of the rectum is to remain empty but in constipation it is nearly always full.

Faeces may be soft, but even soft faeces may not be soft enough. You may feel 'rabbit droppings' even though they were not mentioned by the patient. Inspection and an attempt to insert a finger will soon detect any anal or rectal disease (see Chapter 19). The examining finger may find a rectal tumour which is hard and usually ulcerated. A sigmoid tumour is often felt through the mucosa as an indistinct mass, although it is impossible to distinguish this from a mass due to diverticular disease.

Sigmoidoscopy may detect a tumour further up, but a persistent examining finger is hard to beat. One of the main uses of sigmoidoscopy is in gathering a further clue for the diagnosis of the irritable bowel syndrome. In this condition insufflation produces pain and usually reproduces the pain the patient has suffered before.

INVESTIGATIONS

If there is the possibility of a malignant lesion in the colon causing the constipation, then futher investigation is indicated. This should be by double-contrast barium enema or, if there is

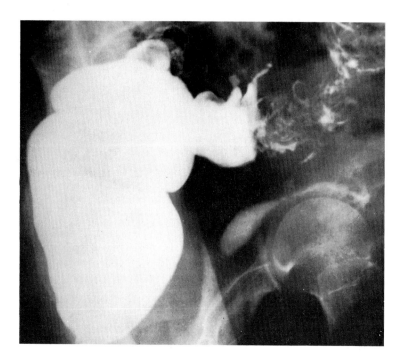

Fig. 18.2 Barium enema showing a stricture in an area of diverticular disease of the colon: benign or malignant?

doubt about the interpretation of the enema, then by colonoscopy. Doubtful areas on the enema are usually the caecum, which may be difficult to distend, and the sigmoid colon. The latter is sometimes difficult to display, but the more common problem is a stricture in an area of diverticular disease; it may be quite impossible to tell from the X-ray film whether it is due to malignancy or not (Fig. 18.2). Unfortunately, colonoscopy in these latter cases is often difficult because the sigmoid colon is stuck down. A successful colonscopy should provide mucosal biopsies from any suspicious areas.

A plasma thyroxine measurement, with or without thyroid-stimulating hormone, will confirm a clinical impression of myxoedema. Similarly, blood levels of potassium and calcium are necessary to exclude rare abnormalities of these cations causing constipation.

There are no other investigations which help. The examination and, most important, the history must give most of the evidence for a confident diagnosis.

MANAGEMENT

Tumours and rarities requiring special investigation and treatment can safely be left to surgeons and other experts. Even if tumours cannot be completely removed and the patient cured, palliation of symptoms is usually possible; removal of the primary colonic cancer, even if there are secondary deposits, is usually wise in order to prevent subsequent obstruction.

We are then left with the vast majority of patients who may be labelled irritable bowel syndrome, diverticular disease, or 'simple constipation', chronic constipation, dyschezia. All of these require some remedy. My preference is for a high-fibre diet. In most people this is quite the most physiological way of approaching the problem and it means that they do not have to take 'medicine'.

Fortunately, high-fibre diets are becoming popular and there are many books on the market which can be recommended to patients: The F-Plan Diet and The F-Plan Calorie and Fibre Chart (Penguin); Fabulous Fibre Cookbook (Pitman); and for diabetics The Diabetics' Diet Book (Martin Dunitz). My patients have gained more from some of these books than from me or the dietitian. However, it is important to spend time talking to the patients about the necessity for the diet. I quote two examples:

A recently retired health professional who had been 'constipated all my life' had never really thought of a high-fibre diet but returned three months later saying 'Now I'm ready for my next sixty years'!

A 25-year-old girl who thought she was on a high-fibre diet came to be investigated because she was certain that her chronic constipation indicated a serious problem. She was unconvinced by my reassurance. A barium enema was clear. She failed to turn up three months later. When written to, she replied that she had read *The F-Plan Diet,* which had convinced her that her previous diet was not good enough. She was so well that she had forgotten her appointment.

The mainstay of all high-fibre diets is an increase in cereal fibre; for most people this means an increase in or an introduction of miller's bran. People's colons are as different from one another as their outward appearance; what is a high-fibre diet for one colon is too much for a second and too little for a third. It is worth stressing this point. Your patient needs a diet sufficiently rich in fibre for him to pass a large soft stool a day: only he can discover for himself how much fibre that means. Most high-fibre diets, having discussed preliminaries and variations in foods, recommend one teaspoonful of bran per day to start with, gradually increasing the dose. Two things are important: firstly, the introduction of dietary fibre must be gradual. Large quantities of bran suddenly appearing in the bowel cause the bacteria to form quantities of gas which distends the abdomen and is anti-social. This leads to demoralisation of patient and doctor:

A lady suffering from the irritable bowel syndrome attended with her husband; I clearly convinced them of the importance of a high fibre intake. They went straight to the nearest health food shop and purchased a generous supply of high-fibre foods. They went home and began to eat them enthusiastically. The inevitable occurred: they were so upset that they did not reappear for two months!

Fibre intake should be increased gradually to the level which produces the desired effect

The second important point is that the intake of fibre must be increased to a level which produces the desired effect. A certain doctor whom I know extremely well consumes nine tablespoons of bran a day. To many this is an enormous amount but it seems right for him.

Many people find miller's bran extremely difficult to eat and it is worth while explaining that it does not have to be eaten neat like a medicine, but can be mixed with any food. It can also be eaten cooked, as well as raw, and this is often more acceptable.

What happens if a high-fibre diet fails? Some patients do not realise that a high-fibre diet is for every day of one's life; it is not to be taken occasionally for acute relief of stubborn bowels. The patient may refuse or be unable to cope with a diet. It is then reasonable to use a proprietary bulking agent for such a patient. There are a large number on the market, made mostly from ispaghula, sterculia or methylcellulose. It is as well to choose one of those that does not contain a stimulant purgative. Similar advice must be given, probably repeatedly, that the appropriate dose is that which produces the desired result. In addition it must be emphasised that these preparations are not designed to be taken intermittently; they should be a permanent treatment for the patient.

There will remain patients who are still not relieved of their constipation; they should be given daily lactulose. Unfortunately, it is so sweet that some patients dislike taking it, but it never fails if the patient will take enough. The dose should be increased slowly, since distension and flatus may again cause problems. Lactulose is a disaccharide which is not absorbed; it is not fattening and can be taken by diabetics.

In general, stimulant purgatives are not advised partly because of their unphysiological nature and partly because they may lead to the condition of 'cathartic colon', when the colon, driven for many years by stimulant purgatives, finally fails to respond. This does not mean that there are not patients for whom stimulatory purgatives are necessary, but they are rare. Patients who have taken stimulant purgatives for years should be given a high-fibre diet, and the purgatives should be withdrawn gradually over a period of months.

> A high-fibre diet is for every day of one's life

FURTHER READING

Burkitt DP (1979) How to manage constipation with a high-fibre diet. Geriatrics 34: 33-40.

Eastwood MA, Passmore R (1983) Dietary fibre. Lancet 2: 202-206.

Leading Article (1980) Investigating constipation. Br Med J 280: 669-670.

Review Article (1981) Wheat bran for diverticular disease. Drug Ther Bull 19: 29-31.

Doctor, I think I've got piles

It is likely that a patient who thinks that anal symptoms are due to 'piles' is entirely correct. It is because most of these patients actually do have 'piles' that a systematic approach is necessary to avoid neglect of other, often more serious, pathology.

The word 'pile' is applied to many normal and abnormal perianal lesions. It is, however, properly used to describe a redundancy of the mucosa of the anal columns overlying the haemorrhoidal plexus; in the interests of precise terminology it is better called a 'haemorrhoid'.

It has for many years been assumed that a haemorrhoid is a form of varicose vein. This is now known to be untrue, the haemorrhoidal vascular plexus being largely irrelevant to the development, symptomatology or treatment of haemorrhoids. A degree of redundancy and laxity of the mucosa of the anal canal is necessary to accommodate the stool during defaecation; it probably also allows discrimination between faeces and flatus. However, if the anal mucosa is forced downwards by straining, the redundancy is increased and the mucosa becomes liable to trauma by the muscles of the anal sphincter. Such trauma results in superficial inflammation with increased production of mucus, which may leak onto the perianal skin, causing irritation or soreness. The inflamed mucosa also bleeds (bright red capillary blood, not the dark blood of varicose veins) and becomes oedematous. The oedematous mucosa within the anal canal may lead a patient to believe that defaecation is incomplete and provoke further straining. If the mucosa becomes sufficiently lax and redundant the patient will eventually become aware of prolapse during defaecation and perhaps find manual replacement necessary. Occasionally replacement is not possible and a painful strangulation results.

It is frequently difficult for patients to appreciate whether or not they are straining excessively on the toilet. Constipation, diarrhoea and unsuccessful attempts at defaecation provoked by inappropriate toilet training or folklore all produce excessive

A haemorrhoid is caused by redundancy of the mucosa of the anal columns overlying the haemorrhoidal plexus

Patients cannot always appreciate whether they are straining unduly on the toilet straining. Many younger patients have a relatively spastic internal anal sphincter muscle which causes additional trauma to the anal mucosa. Gravity may also play a part, the perusal of newspapers and magazines for prolonged periods of time whilst seated on the toilet (an almost uniquely male phenomenon) aggravates mucosal descent. Finally there can be little doubt that even a normal excretory effort will, after many years, result in some degree of prolapse. Thus haemorrhoids are almost invariable in the very elderly, but often cause no symptoms since the anal sphincter is lax.

DIFFERENTIAL DIAGNOSIS

Table 19.1 Differential diagnosis of 'piles'

Fissure in ano
Anterior mucosal prolapse
Perianal haematoma
Fibroepithelial polyps
Skin tags
External haemorrhoids
Proctitis
Carcinoma of rectum or anal canal
Perianal warts
Perianal abscess or fistula
Crohn's disease
Adenomatous or juvenile polyps
Rectal prolapse
Perianal descent and strain

Several common anorectal conditions may give symptoms commonly associated with haemorrhoids.

FISSURE IN ANO. Most fissures occur at the anal margin in the mid-posterior position. They frequently bleed and are very painful. Because a fissure causes spasm of the anal sphincter, the patient may also complain of symptoms from pre-existing but previously symptomless haemorrhoids. However, the characteristic severe pain of a fissure usually indicates the primary cause of the problem. Most fissures can be seen by gently parting the anal opening manually, a manoeuvre which may spare the patient painful instrumentation (Fig. 19.1).

ANTERIOR MUCOSAL PROLAPSE. In some patients the rectal mucosa may prolapse in the midline anteriorly (Fig. 19.2). Such prolapse is particularly common in elderly women; a lax anal sphincter and weakness of the pelvic floor are as important a cause as straining. The symptoms are identical to those of haemorrhoids but the distinction is not entirely academic as, in contrast to haemorrhoids, surgical excision is simple and painless.

PERIANAL HAEMATOMA. Opinion differs as to whether the perianal blood clot is the result of a ruptured perianal vein or thrombosis within the vein ('thrombosed pile'). In either case the result is a discoloured, painful swelling of sudden onset at the external edge of the anus (Fig. 19.3).

FIBROEPITHELIAL POLYPS. Intermittent prolapse of haemorrhoids over many years, in the presence of a spastic anal sphincter, often results in scarring and fibrosis of the haemorrhoid. Continued excessive straining causes the fibrotic nodule to descend further, pulling a mucosal stalk behind it. Eventually this fibrous polyp passes out of the anal canal (Fig. 19.4) and requires manual replacement after defaecation.

SKIN TAGS. The origin of these very common lesions (Fig. 19.5) is uncertain. Sometimes they follow a perianal haematoma or thrombosis and strangulation of haemorrhoids, especially if the prolapse is sufficient to include skin. By impairing effective perianal hygiene the skin tags may be associated with irritation and soreness. Occasionally they are torn during the passage of a constipated stool or after aggressive attempts at cleaning. They then become painful and swollen, or bleed.

EXTERNAL HAEMORRHOIDS. This term is often applied to a variety of perianal lesions. It is best confined to the cutaneous element of a haemorrhoid which is incorporated into the prolapse when the mucosal element is large (Fig. 19.6). The external haemorrhoid is commonly seen when the anal sphincter is relatively lax and remains prominent when the internal haemorrhoid is manually replaced.

PROCTITIS. Inflammatory bowel disease is often confined to the lower rectal mucosa and the mucosal inflammation will produce identical symptoms to haemorrhoids with the exception of prolapse. However, as many of these patients will also have haemorrhoids, the precise cause of their symptoms can be very uncertain.

CARCINOMA. A carcinoma of either the rectum or the anal canal can precisely reproduce the symptoms of haemorrhoids. Carcinoma of the anal canal may often be seen on careful inspection (Fig. 19.7). Either type of carcinoma can always be felt if systematic digital palpation of the rectal mucosa is performed. A barium enema is no substitute for such an examination as, owing to the position of the enema tube, low carcinomas are rarely demonstrated by the radiologist.

PERIANAL WARTS. Most, but not all, perianal warts or condylomata are venereal, and may be associated with other venereal diseases (Fig. 19.8). They may cause extensive irritation and bleed following local trauma.

PERIANAL ABSCESS AND FISTULA. Perianal cellulitis may produce a tender swelling at the anal margin and is particularly painful during defaecation (Fig. 19.9). Insomnia, relieved only by analgesics, is a reliable indication of abscess formation.

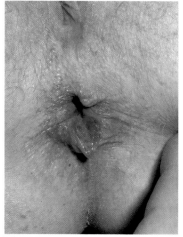

Fig. 19.1 An anal fissure revealed by parting the anal opening.

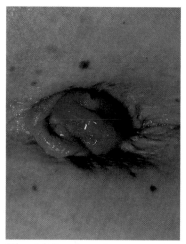

Fig. 19.2 Anterior mucosal prolapse.

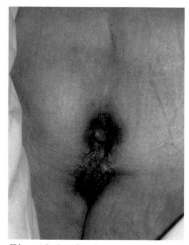

Fig. 19.3 Perinanal haematoma.

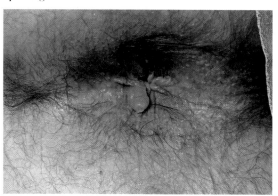

Fig. 19.4 A fibroepithelial polyp prolapsing through the anal canal.

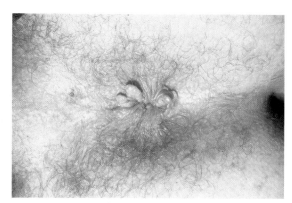

Fig. 19.5 Anal skin tags.

Surgical drainage or spontaneous rupture may be followed by a fistula (Fig. 19.10) which, though painless, discharges on to the perianal skin with resultant soreness and irritation.

CROHN'S DISEASE. Approximately 30% of patients with Crohn's disease present initially with anorectal problems. The typical oedematous skin tags, fissures and fistulae may produce symptoms typical of haemorrhoids, but the difference is easily appreciated by looking at the perineum (Fig. 19.11).

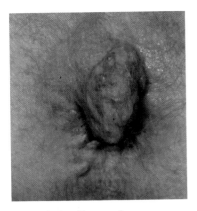

Fig. 19.6 External haemorrhoids.

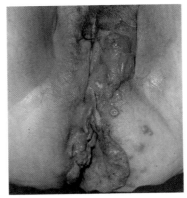

Fig. 19.7 Carcinoma of the anal canal.

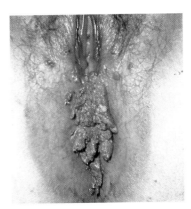

Fig. 19.8 Perinanal warts.

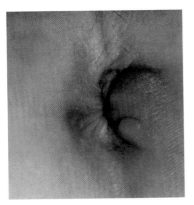

Fig. 19.9 A perianal abscess.

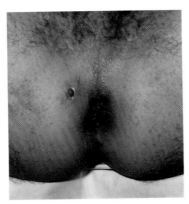

Fig. 19.10 A fistula in ano.

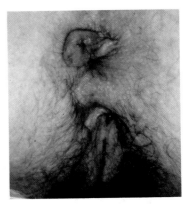

Fig. 19.11 Crohn's disease, with skin tags, a fissure and fistulae.

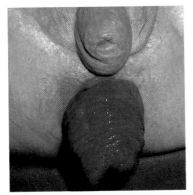

Fig. 19.12 Vaginal and rectal prolapse.

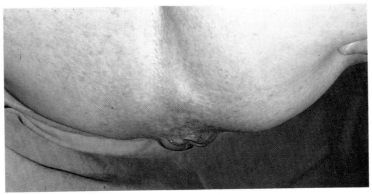

Fig. 19.13 Perineal descent and strain.

ADENOMATOUS AND JUVENILE POLYPS. Much less frequent than fibroepithelial polyps, these lesions may descend through the anal sphincter during defaecation.

RECTAL PROLAPSE. Full-thickness rectal prolapse is rare but occurs most commonly in nulliparous women. The massive prolapse is easily traumatised by underclothes and mucous discharge and bleeding occurs (Fig. 19.12). Incontinence is also common. The prolapse may occur only with defaecation and diagnosis may then be difficult, as these elderly ladies may be naturally reluctant to exert sufficient expulsive effort to produce the prolapse in the surgery.

PERINEAL DESCENT AND STRAIN. Prolonged straining on the lavatory over many years may result in stretching and descent of the pelvic floor (Fig. 19.13). If the sphincter is lax prolapse or incontinence may occur. Much more commonly the sphincter tone remains good and a painful perineal strain results. The pain is usually maximal at the end of the day, or after standing for prolonged periods, as well as after defaecation. There is often no pain on waking in the morning. These patients frequently also have some degree of anterior mucosal prolapse or haemorrhoids, so that diagnosis may be very difficult. However, gentle pressure on the perineal muscles between thumb externally and finger within the rectum will usually localise the source of the pain. Many patients will improve or be cured if straining ceases, but some patients find this very difficult.

CLUES FROM THE HISTORY

The symptoms of haemorrhoids occur in many common anorectal conditions, particularly those in which inflamed or prolapsing anal mucosa is the primary cause. The most detailed history may, therefore, indicate only the approximate anatomical site of the problem and any attempt at diagnosis is dependent on a proper examination.

Diagnosis always depends on a proper examination

There are, however, occasions when the facilities for such an examination are inadequate or the patient may refuse it; in such circumstances (which should be extremely rare) some indication of the possible diagnosis and urgency of further management may be obtained from the history.

Onset

Haemorrhoids may give symptoms from the second decade

onwards. Although younger children may be affected, anal fissures, juvenile polyps and Crohn's disease are more common. The development of haemorrhoids is usually a gradual process, unless prolapse and strangulation are provoked by an acute underlying event such as severe constipation or pregnancy.

Pain

Haemorrhoids, though often sore, are usually not frankly painful unless strangulated and/or thrombosed. Anal fissures, perianal haematoma, abscess, perianal strain and a carcinoma that has invaded the perianal skin are all common causes of perianal pain. The latter possibility demands urgent referral if pain makes adequate examination impossible.

Perianal irritation (pruritus)

A common but by no means invariable symptom, this usually occurs early in the development of haemorrhoids. Inadequate hygiene (sometimes associated with perianal skin tags), specific dermatological disease due to contact sensitivity to 'soothing' creams, fungal infections, threadworms and indeed any cause of rectal or vaginal discharge may provoke such irritation, but haemorrhoids, sometimes only very small, are the commonest cause of pruritus ani.

Bleeding

The bright red blood from surface capillaries of inflamed prolapsing mucosa is characteristic of haemorrhoids, but is equally common in proctitis, anal fissure, anterior mucosal prolapse or carcinoma. Bleeding may only be apparent to the patient with haemorrhoids when seen on the toilet paper after unintentional replacement of the prolapse during cleansing. Depending on the expulsive effort and strangulating effect of the sphincter muscle quite large amounts of blood may be lost into the toilet. Occasionally severe iron deficiency anaemia may result but this should always provoke a search for a colonic carcinoma which is a much more likely cause. Similarly the passage of dark blood or blood mixed with the stools is most unlikely to be due to haemorrhoids and these patients should be assumed to have a carcinoma until proved otherwise.

Colonic carcinoma is a much more likely cause for iron-deficiency than haemorrhoids

Prolapse

Although it is now accepted that some degree of haemorrhoidal prolapse precedes the development of any symptoms, patients do not become aware of this symptom until late in the development of the condition. Initially the prolapse may cause a sensation of incomplete defaecation (tenesmus) or a persistent desire to defaecate which often provokes frequent straining and thus makes matters worse. Patients may also complain that cleaning is difficult. Larger amounts of prolapse are recognised as such but few patients can identify the nature of the prolapse which may be a polyp, anterior mucosal prolapse, rectal prolapse or haemorrhoids. Carcinomas rarely prolapse but frequently cause tenesmus.

ABNORMALITIES ON EXAMINATION

Abdomen

The abdomen should always be examined first as symptoms attributed to haemorrhoids may be due to carcinoma of the colorectum or inflammatory bowel disease.

Anus and rectum

Gentle systematic examination is essential for accurate diagnosis. It is essential to give a reassuring commentary and explanation of precisely what is being done as the examination proceeds. Preparation is unnecessary for digital examination and proctoscopy, but if sigmoidoscopy is planned the bowel may first be emptied by means of a glycerine suppository or phosphate enema.

There are four steps to careful examination of the anus and rectum:

INSPECTION. If internal haemorrhoids are prolapsed, or associated with significant external haemorrhoids, they will be easily seen. Internal haemorrhoids are otherwise not visible at this stage, though they may be indicated by the presence of perianal erythema, excoriation or scratch marks as a result of pruritus. Persistent excessive straining may be inferred from perineal descent below the level of the ischial tuberosity. Inspection of the perianal skin allows skin tags to be seen. It is important to appreciate the significance of the midline posterior skin tag, or 'sentinel pile', which is frequently associated with an underlying anal fissure. A painful digital examination may then be avoided.

PALPATION. Digital examination is best performed wearing a polythene glove which allows maximal sensitivity of the exploring finger. It should be well lubricated with K-Y Jelly. The pulp of the right index finger is placed on the anal opening; gentle and progressive pressure is exerted. This will cause the sphincter to relax even in the most anxious or reluctant patient. Hurried attempts at digital insertion have the opposite effect. On insertion of the finger an attempt is made to assess anal sphincter tone and the anal canal is then explored. The rectum is entered and the mucosal surface palpated. Internal haemorrhoids, unless thrombosed or extremely large, cannot usually be felt. Finally, the cervix, uterus and prostate are assessed and any abnormality of the pelvis or presacral space is detected.

PROCTOSCOPY (Fig. 19.14). Either disposable plastic proctoscopes or the St Mark's Hospital stainless steel type may be used. The stainless steel proctoscope reflects light into the anal canal and allows the use of an Anglepoise type of light, or powerful torch, when necessary. The well-lubricated proctoscope is held lightly by the handle with the thumb holding the obturator firmly in place. With the handle in the midline posteriorly, the tip of the obturator is placed against the anal opening and aimed towards the umbilicus. Pressure is

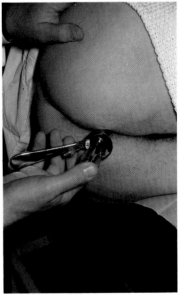

Fig. 19.14 Proctoscopy.

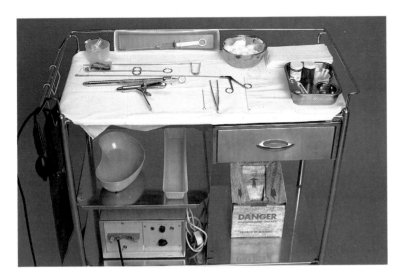

exerted gently and progressively until the sphincter relaxes, when the proctoscope passes into the anal canal. The obturator is removed and the proctoscope held in place with the left hand, the right being free to insert one or two pieces of cotton wool into the rectum using Emmet's forceps. The cotton wool acts as a plug and a reflector of light and need not be removed if the patient is informed accordingly. The rectal mucosa should be inspected and the proctoscope then slowly removed. As it passes through the anal canal the anal columns appear. If abnormally prominent or prolapsing into the proctoscope, a diagnosis of internal haemorrhoids is made. It is often possible to see bleeding from the excoriated mucosal surface of the haemorrhoids as the proctoscope is withdrawn.

SIGMOIDOSCOPY. Sigmoidoscopy allows a direct view of any rectal lesions palpated on digital examination and beyond reach of the proctoscope. It requires more equipment and is more time-consuming than is generally acceptable to a busy general practioner. The examination is not essential for the presumptive diagnosis of rectal carcinoma which should be readily palpable. Rectal biopsy is usually best carried out in hospital where facilities for coping with occasional complications are more readily available.

MANAGEMENT

There has, in recent years, been much controversy over the extent to which surgical treatment is appropriate in the management of haemorrhoids. The account given here is, therefore, a personal view, though it forms a useful basis for staging and treatment.

Stage I haemorrhoids cause perianal irritation, tenesmus, difficulty in cleaning, discomfort and bleeding

Stage I haemorrhoids

Patients complain of perianal irritation, tenesmus, difficulty in cleaning, discomfort or bleeding.

TREATMENT IN GENERAL PRACTICE. Suppositories containing anti-inflammatory steroids and local anaesthetic preparations such as Anusol or Proctosedyl are often effective. In the absence of any bacteriological evidence, local antibiotics or antifungal ointments should be avoided as they frequently cause hypersensitivity rashes.

Treat any constipation with bulk preparations, though stimulant aperients may be necessary.

Advise against prolonged straining, undue expulsive efforts and prolonged perusal of periodicals whilst seated on the toilet. The patient should avoid application of antiseptic or deodorant preparations, either directly to the perianal skin or in the bath or underclothes. Undue vigour in the use of toilet paper is also best avoided; the use of moist paper or if possible a bidet is better.

The patient should always be advised to return for further review if the symptoms do not resolve; this should include a repeat examination. If no explanation for continued symptoms is apparent, referral to hospital is advisable.

TREATMENT IN GENERAL PRACTICE OR IN HOSPITAL. At this stage a sigmoidoscopy should be performed to eliminate small or high rectal lesions that might have been missed on digital examination.

Injection of 5% phenol in vegetable oil is a traditional and well-proved treatment. The injections produce an inflammatory reaction deep to the mucosa above the haemorrhoid and this is followed by a scar which contracts and lifts the lax haemorrhoidal mucosa into the upper anal canal, away from trauma by the anal sphincter. A few patients will experience some discomfort about half an hour after injection but this usually settles after approximately four hours. An injection given too superficially often produces a mucosal ulcer which may bleed until healed. Injections should not be given to patients with an impaired immune response as there is a risk of septicaemia. It is also probably unwise to use this method in patients with Crohn's disease as the injections may provoke exacerbation of the disease.

Whilst the results of injections, banding and cryotherapy are comparable, the author's practice is to treat Stage I haemorrhoids that have failed to respond to adequate management by the patient's general practitioner with injections of phenol in oil. Injections are easy to give, require no skilled assistance, are rarely painful and only exceptionally result in complications.

Application of rubber (Baron's) bands has become very popular in some centres; it is a reasonable alternative to injections. The bands are applied with a special applicator and they strangulate the mucosa, which then sloughs to leave a small scar which draws up the redundant mucosa. The method is rather less messy than injection therapy, but it requires relatively skilled assistance. It may be very painful if low anal mucosa or skin is included in the band. Haemorrhage is the only important complication.

Cryotherapy may be applied with a cryoprobe cooled with liquid nitrous oxide or liquid nitrogen. An assistant is required to hold a plastic proctoscope in place so that freezing of each haemorrhoid can be accomplished without freezing the mucosa on the opposite rectal wall. Although symptomatic relief is usually as good with cryotherapy as after banding or injections, it is often more painful than the other two methods. The ulcers resulting from cryotherapy take a long time to heal, so pain may last up to six weeks.

Stage II haemorrhoids

Stage II haemorrhoids prolapse after defaecation

Patients may complain of any of the symptoms of Stage I haemorrhoids but in addition they are aware of prolapse after defaecation. Spontaneous reduction occurs.

TREATMENT IN GENERAL PRACTICE. All the measures recommended for Stage I haemorrhoids may be considered. Many patients will be quite satisfied if they are free of bleeding, discomfort and pruritus and may be willing to tolerate the occasional prolapse if operation can thereby be avoided.

TREATMENT IN HOSPITAL. The methods previously described may be attempted, but none gives good results with larger haemorrhoids. Only injections of phenol in oil are unlikely to cause complications. If the results of injection are unsatisfactory, the patient will need a surgical procedure.

Maximal anal dilatation to six or eight fingerbreadths will circumferentially stretch the internal sphincter without damaging the external sphincter. The reduced sphincter tone will allow defaecation without excessive effort; any prolapse will undergo less trauma and will reduce more easily. In addition, the submucosal haematoma that follows this procedure will later organise and tend to tether the prolapsing haemorrhoids higher in the anal canal.

This procedure must be performed under general anaesthesia, as it is otherwise very painful; it may provoke cardiac arrhythmia. If proper selection of patients is made, about 90% may expect to be relieved of all symptoms in the short term though long-term results are less certain. Incontinence has been reported after maximal anal dilatation and certain contraindications to the procedure are now recognised. The method should never be applied to the elderly or to patients who have undergone previous operation or suffered injury to their anal sphincter, whose symptoms are not adequately explained by haemorrhoids, or who have a tendency to diarrhoea.

Haemorrhoidectomy may be indicated if symptoms are severe and the patient is not suitable for maximal anal dilatation.

Stage III haemorrhoids

These patients have the characteristic symptoms of haemorrhoids but the prolapse requires manual replacement not only after defaecation but often also after any form of exercise.

Stage III haemorrhoids require manual replacement after defaecation or exercise

TREATMENT IN HOSPITAL. It is often worthwhile giving a set of injections as, although unlikely to give complete resolution of symptoms, they may reduce symptoms to an acceptable level.

Maximal anal dilatation gives remission of bleeding and discomfort in most suitable patients; however, the prolapse may be unaffected and sometimes becomes worse. About 80% of patients will obtain sufficient improvement for further treatment to be unnecessary; a few will return with further symptoms over the subsequent five years and will require haemorrhoidectomy.

Haemorrhoidectomy, once a common operation on any operating list, is now reserved for those patients with large prolapsing haemorrhoids who do not respond to, or are unsuitable for, any other form of treatment. Good judgement is required to remove sufficient mucosa to prevent prolapse and associated haemorrhoidal symptoms, but not so much that excess scarring will lead to an anal stricture. This complication provokes further straining and recurrent symptoms. Haemorrhage both immediate and delayed, faecal impaction and pain are the main postoperative problems. Whilst incontinence is rare, removal of the haemorrhoidal mucosa often impairs sensation. This may make discrimination between flatus and faeces impossible; proper control of flatus may thus become difficult. The unpleasantness of this somewhat infamous operation may be minimised by careful attention to postoperative care. Restriction of the procedure to those with severe symptoms unresponsive to other methods usually ensures a satisfied patient.

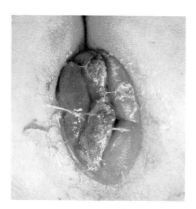

Fig. 19.15 Strangulated haemorrhoids.

Strangulated haemorrhoids

Occasionally the haemorrhoidal mucosa will prolapse after defaecation and the patient will be unable to replace the haemorrhoid. Venous return from the haemorrhoidal plexus is impaired and the haemorrhoids become engorged, oedematous and painful. Thrombosis of the haemorrhoidal plexus may then occur, resulting in necrosis (Fig. 19.15).

TREATMENT IN GENERAL PRACTICE OR HOSPITAL. The patient is confined to bed with the foot of the bed elevated 30 cm or more. A lukewarm bath (with a tablespoonful of salt added) is refreshing; 'ice packs' (the sealed cooling bags for portable cool storage containers are very suitable) reduce the oedema and are soothing. 5% xylocaine ointment may be applied locally, but some form of oral analgesia (paracetamol is least constipating) is usually necessary during the day. A parenteral opiate may be required to prevent insomnia. Aperients will be necessary to allow a soft well-lubricated stool; lactulose is particularly suitable. Resolution is almost invariable and commences about four to five days after strangulation. There is usually little discomfort after 10 days unless extensive necrosis has occurred and then the slough will eventually separate with ulceration and some bleeding. Occasionally, when necrosis is minimal, the haemorrhoid will rupture with drainage of a submucosal haematoma. This is alarming to the patient but results in prompt symptom relief.

TREATMENT IN HOSPITAL. Maximal anal dilatation may give almost immediate relief to patients with strangulated and thrombosed haemorrhoids. The same considerations and contra-indications apply as when used in the absence of strangulation. Haemorrhoidectomy is rarely required.

FURTHER READING

Alexander-Williams J. The management of piles. Br Med J 1982: 385; 1064-1065, 1137-1139.

Alexander-Williams J. Pruritus ani. Br Med J 1983: 287; 159-160.

Editorial (1981) Piles and their P values. Lancet 2: 77.

Index

Abdominal enlargement **125-136**
Abdominal pain
  acute **77-96**
  chronic **67-76**, 172
Abscess
  amoebic liver 113, 115, 122
  perianal 158, 239
Achalasia 12, 16, 21, 24
Addison's disease 168
Aerophagia 71, 220
Albumin infusion 134
Alcohol-related disorders 54, 221
  abdominal pain 70
  diarrhoea 167, 170
  dyspepsia 27, 30
  jaundice 100, 109, 110
  liver enlargement 114
  vomiting 43
  wind 221, 222
  see also Cirrhosis
Alpha-l-antitrypsin deficiency 99
Aluminium hydroxide 221, 230
Amiloride 131, 132
Amitriptyline 76, 220
Amoebiasis 158, 160, 175, 195, 208
Amoebic liver abscess 113, 115, 122
Amphotericin B 221
Ampicillin 94, 164, 208
Amyloidosis 140, 144, 148
Anaemia 32, 61, 102, 113, 139, 144, 157, 202, **211-217**
Anaesthetics, local, for piles 246
Aneurysm 51, 54, 67, 79, 90, 95
Antacids 220
  causing diarrhoea 154, 167
  duodenal ulcer 36
  heartburn 8
Antibiotics
  acute diarrhoea 164
  causing gastrointestinal upset 153, 154, 195, 221
  peritonitis 135
  prophylaxis for gut surgery 94

Antidepressants 76, 230
Antidiarrhoeals 163, 181
Antiemetics 49
Antihistamines 49
Antispasmodics 76
Appendicitis 77, 78, 84, 90, 91
Ascites 110, **125-136**, 221
Azathioprine 109, 209

Baron's bands 247
Belching 27, 71, 220
Bendrofluazide 131
Bethanecol 8
Bilirubin metabolism 97
Biopsy
  gastric ulcer 39
  haematemesis 58
  heartburn 6
  jejunal 178, 192
  liver 107, 119, 120, 149
  rectal 160, 204
  small bowel 160
Bismuth 220
Bloating 224
Bowel
  balloon distension 75
  obstruction 67, 77, 93
  vascular insufficiency 27, 30, 95, 155, 201
Brain stem artery disease 12
Bronchial carcinoma 12, 17
Brucellosis 139, 141
Budd-Chiari syndrome 126
Bulking agents 235, 247
Bumetanide 131

Campylobacter infections 152, 160, 164, 194, 200, 204, 208
Candidiasis 12, 17, 19
Carbenoxolone 8, 39, 220
Carbon tetrachloride causing jaundice 100
Carcinoid 155, 168
Cardiac failure 113, 114, 126
Cardiac ischaemia 1, 27, 28, 67

Caries 224
Carotenaemia 97
CAT scan 90, 129
Cephalosporins 94, 195
Cervical osteophytes 12, 17
Chagas' disease 16
Chenodeoxycholate 40, 220
Chloramphenicol 164, 195
Chlorpromazine 100, 221
Chlorothiazide 131
Cholangiocarcinoma 126
Cholecystitis 77, 84, 91
Cholera 152
Cholestyramine 181, 208, 221
Cimetidine 155, 181, 220
  duodenal ulcer 36
  gastric ulcer 39
  heartburn 8
  peptic stricture 23
Cinnarizine 49
Cirrhosis 99, 109, 113, 114, 121, 128, 130
  see also Ascites *and* Portal hypertension
Clindamycin causing colitis 153, 195
Clofibrate causing diarrhoea 155
Clostridium difficile infection 153, 160, 164, 204, 208
Clostridium welchii infection 153, 160, 164
Codeine phosphate 163
Coeliac disease 70, 161, 168, 182, 212, 221
Colestipol 208
Colonic carcinoma 30, **155**, 158, 160, 185, **200**, 210, 223, 230
Constipation 67, 80, 84, 224, **229-235**
Contraceptive pill 41, 100
Cortical inhibition 18
Corticosteroids 181, 208, 246
Cotrimoxazole 164, 195, 208
Cow's milk allergy 190
Coxsackie infections 79

Crohn's disease   67, 85, 93, 156,
    158, 160, 161, **167, 170, 181,**
    185, 198, 200, 205, 209, 240
Crosby capsule   161
Cryotherapy   248
Cyanocobalamin   216
Cystic fibrosis   168
Cystitis   77, 80
Cytology, oesophageal   22
Cytotoxic drugs causing jaundice
    100

Dehydration   157, 159, 162, 202
Dermatomyositis   12
Diabetes mellitus   79, 168
Diarrhoea
    acute   **151-165**
    bloody   **193-210**
    chronic   **167-182**
    travellers'   154
Diazepam   221
Dicyclomine   76, 220, 221
Diet   69, 97
    acute diarrhoea   163
    causing anaemia   211
    and constipation   229, 230
    duodenal ulcer   36
    elimination   187
    gluten-free   182
    heartburn   7
    high-fibre   76, 181, 187, 224,
        233
    sodium-restricted   130, 133
    vegetarian   211
    and wind   224
Digoxin causing gastrointestinal
    upset   155, 221
Diloxanide furoate   208
Dimethicone   221
Diphenoxylate   163
Diplococcus pneumoniae   135
Diuretics   110, 131
Diverticular disease of colon   2,
    67, 200, 210, 230
Diverticulitis   77, 80, 156
Diverticulosis   168
Drugs causing gastrointestinal
        upsets
    diarrhoea   154, 167
    gastrointestinal haemorrhage   54
    jaundice   99, 109
    tablets causing dysphagia   18
    vomiting,   41, 42, 49
    wind   221
    see also specific agent
'Dry heaves'   43
Duodenal ulcer   27, 28, 36, 51, 52
Duodenitis   221

Dysmenorrhoea   85
Dyspepsia   *see* Heartburn
Dysphagia   2, **11-25,** 41

Eder-Peustow dilatation   23
Encephalopathy, hepatic   122
Endocarditis, bacterial   138, 139,
    141, 147
Endoscopic oesophageal dilatation
    9, 23
Endoscopic retrograde cholangio-
    pancreatography   36, 106
Endoscopic sclerotherapy   63
Endoscopy
    chronic abdominal pain   75
    diarrhoea   177, 206
    dysphagia   20, 22
    haematemesis   56, 58, 61
    heartburn   6
    indigestion   35
    vomiting   47
Entamoeba histolytica   115, 152, 158
Erythema   172, 201, 203
Erythromycin   164, 208
Escherichia coli   135, 160, 164

Faecal impaction   158
Faeces, examination   158, 174,
    186, 204
Familial Mediterranean fever   67
Felty's syndrome   143,144
Ferrous sulphate causing jaundice
    100
Fibroids   78, 85, 90, 95
Filariasis   126
Fissure, perianal   158, 202, 238
Fistula
    gastrocolic   155, 224
    perianal   202, 239
Food
    allergy   69, **183-192**
    relationship to abdominal pain
        69, 70
    see also Diet
Frusemide   131, 132

Gallstones   2, 27, **29, 40,** 67, 74,
    78, 90, 99, 101, 122, 224
Gastric carcinoma   27, 29, 39, 41,
    51, 54, 223
Gastric ulcer   27, 28, 39, 51, 52,
    85
Gastrinoma   155
Gastritis   41, 42, 49, 221
Gastroenteritis   77, 80, 84, 85,
    153, 154, 161
Gastro-oesophageal reflux   *see*
    Heartburn

Gaucher's disease   139, 140, 144,
    148
Gentamicin   94
Giardiasis   153, 158, 160, 161,
    164, 175
Gilbert's syndrome   98, 105, 108
Glucose tolerance test   178
Goitre, retrosternal   12, 17
Gout   143
Granulomatous disease of liver
    126

Haemangioma   51
Haematemesis   45, **51-65**
Haematological investigations
    acute abdominal pain   88
    anaemia   214
    chronic abdominal pain   73
    diarrhoea   159, 174, 204
    dysphagia   20
    enlarged liver   117
    haematemesis   56
    indigestion   32
    splenomegaly   145, 146
    vomiting   46
Haematoma
    epigastric   80
    perianal   238
Haemochromatosis   115
Haemoglobinuria, paroxysmal
    nocturnal   67
Haemolysis, excessive   98, 140
Haemorrhage, gastrointestinal
    51-65, 77, 80, 114, 211
    see also Haematemesis *and*
    Melaena
Haemorrhagic telangiectasia   51
Haemorrhoids   *see* Piles
Halothane causing jaundice   100
Heartburn   **1-9,** 28, 44, 67, 84,
    211
Henoch-Schönlein purpura   126
Hepatitis   79, 98, **99, 108,** 113,
    114, **122,** 138, 139, 141, 144,
    146
Hepatitis B antigen   57, 63, 98,
    119
Hernia
    hiatus   9, 15, 22, 28, 41, 53, 84,
        221, 222
    strangulated   80
    umbilical   126
Herpes zoster   79
Hirschsprung's disease   230
Hydatid cysts   113, 115, 122, 138,
    139
Hydrochlorothiazide   131
Hyoscine   220

Hypercalcaemia   41, 42
Hyperemesis gravidarum   42
Hypoalbuminaemia   126
Hypothyroidism   126
Hypovolaemia   60

Ibuprofen   189
Ileitis   77, 80, 84
Imipramine   76, 220
Indigestion   see Diarrhoea,
    Heartburn, Wind etc.
Infections
    causing acute abdomen   77
    causing diarrhoea   152, 185
    causing splenomegaly   138
Infectious mononucleosis   79, 98,
    138, 139, 141, 144, 146
Intestinal angina   67, 70
Intussusception   78, 95
Iron therapy   62
Irritable bowel syndrome   1, 27,
    30, **67-76**, 80, 156, 169,
    179-181, 185, 225, 229
Ischaemic colitis   198, 209
Ispaghula   235

Jaundice   **97-111**

Kala azar   138, 139, 142, 147
Kaolin and morphine   163
Ketoacidosis   79
Ketokonazole   221
Kidney stones   78, 95

Lactose intolerance   69, 175, 221,
    222
Lactulose   235, 250
Laparoscopy   120
Laparotomy
    acute abdomen   89, 90, 92, 93
        94, 96
    haematemesis   60
    jaundice   108
Laxative abuse   154, 168, 230
Lead poisoning   67, 79
Leukaemia   113, 126, 139, 141
    144, 147
LeVeen shunt   134
Lincomycin   153, 181, 195
Liquorice   220
Liver
    abscess   113, 115, 122
    enlarged   **113-123**
    malignancy   113, 114, 121, 126
    palpation   102
    see also Cirrhosis and Jaundice
Liver fluke infection   123
Loperamide   163, 181

Lorazepam   221
Lupus erythematosus   126, 139,
    143, 144, 148
Lymphoma   126, 139, 144, 148

Malaria   138, 139, 142
Mallory Weiss tear   45, 51, 53,
    58
Malnutrition   126
Mebeverine   76, 221
Mediastinal tumour   126
Mefenamic acid   167
Meig's syndrome   126
Melaena   158, 175, 212, 243
Menstruation and abdominal pain
    70
Mesenteric adenitis   80, 85
Methylcellulose   235
Methyldopa   100, 155
Metoclopramide   8, 50, 221
Metronidazole   94, 122, 164, 181,
    208, 224
Mianserin   76
Migraine   41, 42
Mittelschmerz   80, 85, 94
Multiple sclerosis   12
Munchausen syndrome   54, 80
Muscular dystrophy   12
Musculoskeletal causes of
    abdominal pain   71, 186
Myasthenia   12
Myelofibrosis   139, 140, 142, 144,
    146
Myeloma   139, 144
Myocardial infarction   79, 221,
    224
Myxoedema   97, 229, 231

Nephrotic syndrome   126
Non-steroidal anti-inflammatory
    drugs   13, 39, 52, 54, 62
Nystatin   221

Oedema, peripheral, with ascites
    128, 132
Oesophageal manometry   6, 22
Oesophageal pH monitoring   6
Oesophageal spasm   12, 16, 21
Oesophageal stricture   3, 12, 21,
    22, 23
Oesophageal varices   51, 54, 62,
    114, 122, 147
Oesophagitis   **1-9**, 12, 51, 53,
    58, 221
    see also Heartburn
Oesophagus
    Barrett's   13, 53
    carcinoma   12, 13, 24, 51

Oesophagus (continued)
    foreign body   12
    haematoma   12
    surgical transection for
        haematemesis   63
    ulcer   12, 18, 51
Ovarian cyst   78, 79, 85, 90, 94
Oxethazaine   220
Oxytetracycline   224

Pancreas
    carcinoma   29, 99, 101, 168
    insufficiency   181
    tests of function   178
Pancreatic enzyme supplements
    181
Pancreatitis
    acute   67, 77, 80, 89, 92, 93,
        125, 126
    chronic   27, 29, 42, 99, 125,
        126, 168
Paracentesis   133
Paracetamol causing jaundice   100
Parkinson's disease   12
Paul Bunnell test   104, 147
Pelvic inflammatory disease
    67, 71
Penicillamine   109, 110
Penicillamine causing diarrhoea
    195
Peppermint   76, 221
Peptic structure   3
Peptic ulcer   1, 41, 62, 67, 70,
    84, 92, 114, 222
    see also Gastric ulcer and
        Duodenal ulcer
Perforation   77, 80
Pericarditis   79
Perineum, descent   242
Peritonitis   127, 135
Perphenazine   49
Pethidine addiction   80
Pharyngeal disorders   11-13
Pharyngeal carcinoma   12, 18
Phenol injection   247
Phenylbutazone causing jaundice
    100
Pica   212
Piles   **237-250**
Pirenzepine   37, 220
Pitressin   63
Pleural effusion   128
Pneumonia   79, 85
Polycythaemia   113, 139, 142
Porphyria   67, 79
Portal hypertension   127, **139,
    144, 147**, 211
Post-gastrectomy syndrome   41

Potassium supplementation   132
Prednisolone   109
Pregnancy   79, 125, 221
    causing vomiting   41, 42
    ectopic   79, 85, 90, 95
Prochlorperazine   49
Proctitis   239
Proctoscopy   73, 173, 245
Propantheline   220
Proptosis   71
Protein-losing enteropathy   73
Pruritus   243
Pseudodysphagia   18
Pseudomembranous colitis   153,
    160, 194, 204, 208
Pseudomyxoma peritonei   126
Pseudoxanthoma elasticum   51
Psychiatric factors in gut disorders
    acute abdomen   67, 68, 69,
        72, 80
    constipation   230
    diarrhoea   171
    dysphagia   18
    spurious gastrointestinal
        haemorrhage   54
    vomiting   41, 42, 43
    wind   221
    see also Irritable bowel syndrome
Pulmonary embolism   79, 85
Purpura, idiopathic
    thrombocytopenic   139, 142
Pyelonephritis   77, 80
Pyloric stenosis   41, 49
Pyoderma gangrenosum   201, 203

Radiology
    acute abdominal pain   88, 90
    chronic abdominal pain   73
    constipation   233
    diarrhoea   160, 161, 175, 176
        177, 205
    dysphagia   20, 22
    enlarged liver   119, 120
    haematemesis   57
    heartburn   5
    indigestion   32
    jaundice   106
    vomiting   47
Radiotherapy   12, 18, 24
Ranitidine   220
    duodenal ulcer   36
    heartburn   8
Rectal carcinoma   84, 158, 239
    ctal examination
        ominal pain   72
        ation   231
        158, 172, 202
    4

Rectal polyps   238, 242
Rectal prolapse   238, 242
Renal calculi   78, 90
Regurgitation   2, 41
Resuscitation, emergency   60
Rheumatoid arthritis   139, 143,
    144, 149
Rotavirus infections   160
Rubber band ligation   247

Salmonella infections   152, 153, 158
    160, 164, 193, 208
Salpingitis   77, 78, 85, 90, 94
Sarcoidosis   139, 143, 149
Schistosomiasis   113
Sclerotherapy   63
Sengstaken-Blakemore tube
    compression   63
Shatski ring   12, 15
Shigella infections   152, 158, 160,
    164, 194, 208
Sickle cell disease   79, 98
Sigmoidoscopy   73, 89, 159, 173,
    204, 232, 246
Skin tags, perianal   158, 202, 238
Skin testing for food allergy   186
Sodium cromoglycate   188, 209
Spherocytosis, hereditary   98
Splenomegaly   137-150
Spironolactone   110, 131, 132, 167
Spleen, ruptured   79, 141
Steatorrhoea   226
Sterculia   235
Sucralfate   37, 220
Sulphasalazine   208, 221
Sulphonamides   94
Surgery
    achalasia   24
    acute abdomen   90, 94, 95, 96
    bowel obstruction   93
    diarrhoea after   168
    duodenal ulcer   38
    gallstones   40, 92
    gastric carcinoma   40
    haematemesis   61
    heartburn   9
    jaundice, obstructive   110
    peptic stricture   23
    perforated peptic ulcer   92
    piles   249, 250
    splenomegaly   150
    vomiting   42
    wind after   221
    see also Laparotomy
Systemic sclerosis   12, 16, 168,
    172

Tabes dorsalis   79
Telangiectasia, haemorrhagic   51
Testicular torsion   80
Tetracycline   100, 164, 181, 195
Thalassaemia   216
Thiotepa   135
Thyroid carcinoma   168
Thyrotoxicosis   168
Trauma   79, 85, 96, 126, 141
Triamterene   131, 132
Trifluoperazine   49
Trimethoprim   94, 164
Trimipramine   220
Tri-potassium di-citrato
    bismuthate   37
Tropical splenomegaly   139
Tropical sprue   160, 161
Trypanosomiasis   138, 139
Tuberculosis   126, 139
Typhoid   139, 142, 144

Ulcer   see Gastric ulcer, Duodenal
    ulcer etc.
Ulcerative colitis   156, 158, 160,
    161, 185, 196, 205, 208
Ultrasound examination   33, 90,
    106, 148
Uraemia   41, 42
Urinary tract infection   94
Ursodeoxycholate   40, 220

Vancomycin   164, 208
Vasculitis   126
Venesection   109
Vestibular disturbances   41, 42
Vibrio cholerae infections   152, 160
Vibrio parahaemolyticus   153, 160,
164
VIPoma   155
Vitamin supplements   110, 216
Volvulus   78, 95
Vomiting   2, 84, 156, 200
    blood   see Haematemesis
    chronic   41-50
Vomitus, inspection of   44

Warts, perianal   239
Whipple's disease   126
Wilson's disease   99, 109
Wind   28, 70, 101, 125, 126,
    219-227

Xylose tolerance test   175

Yersiniosis   153, 160

Zollinger-Ellison syndrome   168